"Average JOE"- *Simple, easy nutrition and exercise plan for you to take with you along life's journey.*

Contents

Dedication

Page

Preface

Dedication

Thank you to God, my beloved family and friends! Without you there could be no me and the realization of my goals!

Preface

This book is intended to help the "Average Joe;" the guy who just wants to live a nice long life with as few health hurdles as possible. Average Joe is meant to be a learning tool to help you start your journey towards better health, no matter at what age you crack open the cover and start to read. If you are before the age of 30 I hope you seriously pay attention and do your best to adhere to the information outlined. If you are reading this book and you older than 30 you can still embed the health information to create that lifestyle you always desired. You are never too old to learn to better improve your health. Use Average Joe to reinforce your daily health habits; an accountability tool. Use Average Joe to guide you towards improved health habits. Use Average Joe to confirm that you are on the right track possibly confirming what you are doing is correct. I have spent the time already combing the research for you. What I have placed in Average Joe is hard science but cut out the "extra fluff" to provide you with the A, B, C's of what you need to do take care of yourself along life's journey.

Let me start off by saying that I am a firm believer, what I think are non-refutable, core facts; in my eyes. This Earth is covered with a plethora of God made vegetation and animals. Most of which are edible in some shape or form and those that are not can serve for other purposes such as for the development of medications, and other uses deemed necessary by humanity. That being said, a basic concept that I and others have conceptualized and believe in is that this Earth will always, if we nurture it, provide our harvest. It will allow you to nurture and thrive as a human being. In regards to nutrition, one would tend to believe that it only makes sense to consume those foods that were put on this Earth; meaning limiting the consumption of man-made foods. This concept will be repeated throughout your reading of this short book. Look, it just makes sense. Without dwelling too much into the science of it, the "goodness" of whole (Earth derived) foods comes from the soil. The soil is where the minerals and other nutrients are found to assist in the optimal growth of the vegetation and animals; so why would it not do the same for you? So, keep nutrition simple and consume from the Earth and limit all man-made processed foods!

The idea of living a long and disease free life has always intrigued me since my early years in college. Throughout my career and travels I have had the opportunity to work with and experience many areas of health care that have led me to write this book. I started with the notion of taking what I know, what the latest research has proven, and a common sense approach, to provide you with what I and others promote the way in which we should take care of our bodies.

The average American male born in 2010 can now expect to live to 76 years (Worldbank, 2012). This is the "average age of no return," keeping in mind that during his life he may endure multiple chronic diseases that will slowly eat away and consume his body until he passes. If lucky, you may only have to endure or experience one or so "bad years" toward the end of your life. However, what is also very plausible is that you could be riddled with disease starting in your twenties or even your teenage years; making the life very burdensome for you and your loved ones. Fear and mental anguish of the sense of mortality would certainly come into the picture if a "stance" is not taken by you. All overweight and obese adults (age 18 years of age or older) with a Body Mass Index (BMI) of 25 or more are considered at risk for developing associated morbidities or diseases such as hypertension, high blood cholesterol, type 2 diabetes, coronary heart disease, and other diseases. Individuals with a BMI of 25 to 29.9 are considered overweight, while individuals with a BMI of 30 are considered obese (What are Overweight and Obesity, NHLBI, 2013). BMI table can be found in the Appendix, page 85. The prevalence of overweight and obesity in adults in the United States increased markedly during the last decade. According to NHANES III data, 54.9 percent of U.S. adults aged 20 years and older are either overweight or obese; 32.6 percent are overweight, defined as having a body mass index (BMI)* of 25.0 to 29.9 kg/m2; and 22.3 percent are obese with a BMI of 30 kg/m2 (CDC, 2012). Type II diabetes and preliminary stages of cardiovascular disease (hypertension-"high blood pressure", hypercholesterolemia-"high cholesterol") can start as early as the pre-teen years ("The Bogalusa Heart Study" (n.d. and Oliveira et al, 2010)). This paves the way as to why men must be visiting their primary care physician or provider (PCP) on an annual basis; *prevention* is a major point in this book. Throughout the book you will note the * and **BOLD** words. These are simply points that must be driven into the man's life; the earlier they are embedded into his life, the better possible outlook. This book is meant to be a common sense approach to optimal health. A prime example of this, to be later detailed, is the human diet. To me, the human diet can be broken down to be made extremely simple. Over the years we have found that what "man" tends to play with, he destroys. Take a very simplistic strategy when following nourishment over your life cycle. "Eat from the ground up!" It is a very elementary style of eating; meaning the less processed by "man," the healthier it will be for you. Sweet and simple! I used to, and still do tell my clients to eat from the earth; vegetables, fruits, and grains. In addition, eat foods that consume sources from the earth; lean meats and dairy. You cannot make it any simpler than that! The closer to earth you consume, the less chance you will have of other processed materials such as chemical dyes, and other flavors, taste or shelf life enhancers that you will be bringing into your body's system. This will provide you with a firm grip on the beginnings of a lifetime of satisfying nourishment for your body. In regards to dietary consumption, from this point on it will simply be a story of how many calories and what type of macronutrients (Carbohydrates, Protein and Fat) to consume. Exercise and physical activity will be detailed in each chapter as well. However, let's take a moment to address this on simple scale. Take a look around and notice how the white collar regime is overcoming the American workplace. We are becoming more and more sedentary in our everyday tasks; technology is killing us faster and faster each day. It takes a "rocket scientist;" (feel the sarcasm), to know that if we do have one of these positions in which we sit or mostly sit for eight to ten hours per day all week, we must alternatively find a way to utilize the calories we consume. If we do not increase our caloric expenditure we will gain the approximate one pound per year for the average American male (Yanovski, J.A., 2000); which unfortunately if not dealt with will expedite chronic disease and lead to a premature death. Therefore, if we do have one of these types of positions at work, we must realize this just means that we have to find a creative way to either decrease calories consumed or increase calories expended. This sounds too easy, and of course for most folks it is probably the hardest venture they will ever take on in life. Regulating and controlling food consumption is very tough for most folks and increasing physical activity/exercise is a close second. So, what are we to do? Literature tells us for best results to focus on both; decreasing calories slowly and increase daily physical activity/exercise. Again, this goes back to embedding this into your daily life; making this an everyday phenomena. So, in theory we need to exercise that much harder and longer and decrease our calories to offset our sedentary workplace. This is challenging because last time I checked, there is still only twenty four hours in a day. Also, in a society that continues to work harder and longer each and every day, we must be creative in the ways in which we approach our "health schedule." Creative ideas, as I will discuss in later chapters is how to get the most "bang for your buck" when it comes to your daily workouts and physical activity. The simplistic way is a must to approach the dietary consumption plan for the human lifecycle. This is something that I have experimented with and have learned and practiced my best each and every day. Like I said, it is not rocket science!

So, once again before we start our voyage towards optimal health, remember, this is meant to be a simplistic journey towards improving your health and never letting it fall back on to the back burner. I cannot lie; it will be very challenging at times especially if you were *not* brought up in a so called "healthy" environment; you start working challenging hours, you get married, you have children, you have too many obligations, et cetera, et cetera, et cetera! Take a moment before we start to recognize the very important point. ***If you do not have your health, you have nothing***!

Men in their 20s- Let's get to know the Basics!

Why should I think early in life about taking care of myself? These are supposed to be my invincible years! I have only lived for twenty some years; I am strong, appear very healthy, can run until my lungs give out! There is absolutely no reason for concern. I am starting my post-school life, my first professional "real" job; I must focus on my career and making my steps count. For I want to be ten steps ahead by the time I reach my late twenties and twenty steps ahead by my early thirties. I must progress forward even if this means sleepless nights, skipping meals, eating more fast food, missing workouts and slightly abusing my overall body functions. I can always take care of my body a little bit later, as I have in the past, it has always bounced back. I am not afraid as I must make my mark on this world first, only then, will I break and focus on me!

I have seen this many, many times, especially in my fellow men that had, in the past, taken care of their bodies. This is unfortunate.

Balance is the key! The earlier you learn that you must take care of your body and balance that with life, the more you will understand that you are now in the "game" of life for the long haul. In addition, you will comprehend and "get" that you MUST have this balance in order to succeed in whatever endeavor (s) you endure whether it is professionally, or socially. You will realize that fueling your body with the right foods, adequate sleep, and getting regular exercise will expedite your success in all areas of your life. You will find that your efforts in all aspects of your life will benefit from the clarity and focus you will receive from taking care of yourself.

A letter to my friends....

My Dear taking over the world good friend,

How do you think the CEOs of major companies have climbed the ladder to their current status? Surely they were not lazy in their efforts. They obviously studied and worked hard in their chosen fields and of course were very driven. However, only those who are truly intuitive to their "self" realize that all their hard work and efforts must pay off! I suppose there are a few that really take care of themselves. For the majority, why would you want to work 12 hour days for 20 some years and die of a heart attack in your early 50's? Or, work so hard and all of sudden wake up at 45 to realize that you are forty pounds overweight, have total blood cholesterol of 300 mg/dl and a resting blood pressure of 160/100? This is a time bomb waiting to explode at such a young age. This never made sense to me. I think there may be more to this life then to work like a dog and then die young or at least become incapacitated to certain degree so that you truly cannot enjoy life! Think about it my young friend. If you do not have your health, all is wasted.

Sincerely,

You, twenty years from now; as I look back in not so good of health! Take the time *NOW* to take care of yourself—if not, you may pay dearly later!

In this book we will keep the word *diet* to mean what you are consuming on a daily basis, *not that you are on a "diet" trying to lose weight.* A diet should advance and evolve with age as you become more able to accept new knowledge and apply to your daily consumption. We will discuss in this chapter the basics of a clean and supportive life cycle diet. You will notice that it will not change much per chapter. Therefore, it is vital that you grasp its importance in the earlier decades of life to reap the long term benefits such as staying lean, healthy (mostly preventative to be disease free), and full of energy. Let's not waste any more time, let's get down to the meat and potatoes of the diet.

Nutrition

First and foremost you must understand the reason for this route of human consumption. The <u>keys to longevity</u> are to stay healthy, and as disease free as possible. Remembering that you should consume most of your diet from the earth (or ground up)! This means, in simple terms, limiting as much as you can the man-made foods. This also means we must present the body with key nutrients that we know prevent diseases. So, let's first introduce the most important, in my eyes, groups of foods to prevent disease and staying lean; vegetables and fruits. Vegetables and fruits are vital players in the longevity of the human body for several reasons. First, collectively, they are naturally the lowest calorie food groups that we can choose on this earth. They are chock full of natural prospective disease fighters, called antioxidants, that can potentially fight against diseases ranging from common colds to diabetes, to cancers (Johnson, 2004). There are several different types, classes, of antioxidants and they are being shown to be the pathway to optimal human health (Appendix, Antioxidants, page 86). Simply put, these naturally food derived fighters are substances that protect your body's cells against the effects of free radicals, aka stress, which infects the human body. Free radicals are molecules that are produced when your body breaks down food, or by environmental exposures such as exposure to tobacco; free radicals can damage cells! Antioxidants may also enhance immune defense and therefore lower the risk of chronic disease. There are also many other nutrients that are important in the vegetable and fruit kingdom. As a side note, since 2005 I have been consuming two mixtures most every morning that I am home and firmly believe they are assisting me in vitality and eventually disease prevention in years to come. In addition, I have yet to truly be sick in over twelve years; a testament to these drinks? I am not certain, but I am at least betting they are assisting in keeping me very healthy! These are both very simple mixes and no need for any mixers or juicers, etc. My first concoction is a garlic, apple cider vinegar and honey mix:

- Purchase a 20-30 oz container.
- No matter what the size it should resemble the following: 1 garlic bulb (minced or at least finely cut); this would equal about 10% of the container, 60% apple cider vinegar, and 30%, 100% raw honey.
- Put in refrigerator and allow mixture to sit for at least a few days prior to using, thus allowing the separate ingredients to infuse with one another.

- In the morning take with breakfast; shake it up a few times, take one "short swig."
- You will taste the acidity of the vinegar but it will be offset by the tad of sweetness from the honey with a touch of garlic.
- It is not bad at all, trust me!

The second concoction is a mix of 100% Pomegranate juice and 100% tomato juice; again combining sweet and salty- offsetting each one's potency:

- Simply "eye" measure one ounce of Pomegranate juice and two ounces of tomato juice and consume.

These two concoctions are providing you with an array of antioxidants first thing in the morning to assist you in fighting your stress and in hopes of preventing chronic diseases in the future.

Fiber is one of the reasons for the lower caloric value and the reason vegetables and fruits are vital attackers against heart disease, cancers and type II diabetes. Men should have on average between 30-35 grams per day according to the Institute on Medicine (Dietary Reference Intakes for Energy, Carbohydrate, Fiber, Fat, Fatty Acids, Cholesterol, Protein, and Amino Acids; Institute on Medicine, 2002).

More fiber should be consumed if you consume more calories. This may prove to be a challenge as most men only consume about 14 grams per day. The recommended amount can easily be consumed if a little bit of planning takes place. It appears to be a challenge to consume that much fiber, especially if you are in the current average group of 14 grams per day. That being said, if we break it down into five feeding times (fancy nutritional jargon for snacks/meals) per day that is only a measly seven grams per meal! Simply remember that you want to consume on average five to nine servings of fruit and vegetables per day. This will lead to a solid foundation and the basic building blocks of the human diet. A simple guide is that a portion size for most vegetables and fruit is about a tennis ball sized serving. *Keep it simple*! Consume what you can on your budget. If you can, eat as much fresh produce as you can; and seasonal produce is always more fiscally sound to purchase. However, if you must consume frozen vegetables; purchasing on sale and storing in the freezer is a great way to keep them available year round. Lastly, if you must, consume canned produce. If canned fruits, certainly drain the excess fluid and purchase in light syrup or natural juices only when you can. If vegetables, purchase the no added salt if you can. If you cannot purchase no added salt versions then strain the can before you eat. The vegetables and fruits are the hardest groups to remember to consume on a daily basis; simply because it is not in our American mindset to consume. We know we should consume them, but we just do not apply. However, by introducing regular vegetable and fruit servings as a part of your stressful and filled 20's decade, you will be setting yourself up to fight many diseases in the duration of your life cycle and assist in reducing your inflammation within your body on a regular basis. In essence, you are betting that they will work in your favor to extend your productive years and beyond! How many do you specifically need at the very least? (Appendix, Fruit and Vegetable amounts per age and activity level, page 91).The vegetarian realm has grown tremendously in the past decade. Long gone are the days of just having tofu for three meals per day. The nutrition companies and grocery stores are catering heavy to the vegetarian audience, thus easing the availability. There are varying types of vegetarianism. A true "vegan," does not eat any animal flesh or byproducts of the animal, for example, milk or eggs, period. There are other types of vegetarianism that are less restrictive. They are Lacto-ovo-vegetarians, who eat both dairy products and eggs; the most common type of vegetarian diet. Lacto-vegetarians eat dairy products but avoid eggs. Ovo-vegetarian, is one who eats eggs but not dairy products. A newer term passing around the vegetarian circles is the pescatarian. This person would not eat land animals but would consume seafood. A vegetarian lifestyle would be optimal way to live if solely focused on health. Vegans would not be consuming the food that leads to clogging your blood vessels; thus almost closing the door to heart attacks and strokes until much later in life. Even at this point it may only be due to a genetic trait. They would also have the easiest time maintaining their weight, as most caloric laden foods come from animals and their byproducts. This would almost close the door on high blood pressure, high cholesterol and type 2 diabetes. If this is something you wish to pursue, make sure you do your research; as sometimes it can be complicated to ensure you are correctly consuming all the vital nutrients you need to nourish your body. If you cannot work with the vegan dietary plan maybe the alternative aforementioned modified versions could work for you? Any of these types of vegetarianism dietary plans can only enhance your health today and in the long run.

The second most important area to consume on a daily basis is lean protein. Your body needs carbohydrates (vegetables, fruit and grains), protein (meats and dairy), and fats (nuts, and primarily oils), to optimally run on a daily basis. The key is to optimize your diet and caloric balance. We have already discussed how to do this with the vegetables and fruits. Now, we must discuss supporting the musculature in the human body, protein. There are many sources of protein, the best being egg whites, animal protein, and soy. That said, the key here is "lean." What does lean mean? It simply means taking in the lowest amount of saturated fat (generally can be interpreted as animal fat, however some other foods in nature do contain) per serving of protein. Egg whites and soy are not the problem here; nor fish or other seafood for the most part. Even so called "fatty fish" are great sources, such as your cold water harvested fish, they contain healthy fat (oil) which they must sustain in the cold depths to keep them alive. The issue comes with the land animals, realizing that most land animals are very large and have many cuts to them. We must be wise as to which cuts of these animals we choose to consume. For the fowl (chicken and turkey) it is best to stick with the breasts. On the cow and the pig, the best to consume are the "loin," and "round" cuts. Most wild animals, such as venison, buffalo, and ostrich are very lean and most of their cuts pass the test as to optimal cuts to consume. We must then discuss preparation. The simplest and healthiest ways to prepare these sources of protein are simply to bake, broil, poach, steam, stir fry or grill. With grilling just be careful not to consume too much of this on a regular basis, especially really charred meats, as current research points to the possibility of causing some types of cancers. A tip to not cooking every night that I have bought into since I was twenty something is to batch cook on a Saturday or Sunday; saving time and effort! I simply just grab my protein portions from the large amount I had cooked on either of these days and always have my meals prepped to go during the week; a great timesaver! This saves a lot of time during the week, as life does tend to get busy especially during the week. It also saves you time not having to cook every night; a tiresome task sometimes after a busy day! In addition, batch cooking allows you to stay on track with your dietary plan as you should not be tempted by other foods because you will not want to waste your money by allowing your meats to spoil. So, how about amount? How much should I consume? I recommend an active man, to be discussed in a bit, to consume a hand sized serving per meal eaten. This should provide you with at least 4-6 servings of lean protein per day; see Appendix, Lean protein list, page 92. Your specific needs will of course be based on your goal. We will discuss this section next after the dietary portion. A preview, though, would be to have a goal of staying "lean" for life; which will entail staying within a five to ten pound weight range of your given adult weight. Of course, if you must lose weight to get down to a "safe" weight for your adulthood, we will discuss that as well. This weight can/should be projected by using BMI. You should try to achieve a healthy BMI, between 18.5 and 24.9 in a perfect world; staying between the targeted five to ten pounds in this range. However, this may be slightly modified when you contact and develop the rapport with your primary care physician (PCP) or provider as he/she may be agreeable to a slightly higher BMI, pending on your internal health. You can be above this BMI and be completely healthy. The healthy BMI range may be a long term target for some; thus the collaborative efforts with your PCP are vital to obtain which may seem like a daunting task. Before the active part of this chapter starts we must move on to the grain world.

Grains, again, with the fruit and some of the higher carbohydrate vegetables, will be the largest source of clean energy for your body to run on. Grains, especially whole grains, have been touted in the news as of the past several years to assist in decreasing your chances of developing heart disease, stomach and bowel cancers, type II diabetes, and weight gain. It is very important to ensure that you are consuming the whole grain; the bran, endosperm, and germ, as they all play vital roles. The bran, is fiber rich and contains a load of B- vitamins and minerals. The endosperm, contains the carbohydrate and protein source of the grain. The germ, contains antioxidants, vitamins E, B and a hint of healthy fat (Appendix, Anatomy of the Whole Grain, page 93). It is recommended that at least half of the grains you consume should come from the whole grain variety (USDA, 2012). I will tell you this, the only grains you should consume, should be whole grains! Though the non-whole grains, often called refined grains, are tempting to want to consume. We know these types of grains commonly as spaghetti, pizza, donuts, cakes, etc in which some of these do actually have whole grain versions; they should only be consumed ever so often such as holidays or special functions. I am all for consuming these types of grains every once in a while to keep sanity and normalcy in a challenging life. That being said, on a daily basis try to ensure that the grains consumed are of the whole grain version. You will need about eight ounces of total grains per day. It is again recommended that at least half come from the whole grain variety. Most Americans, in general, have a challenging time incorporating whole grains into their daily consumption. One phrase, do not be one of them! It takes a tad of work to incorporate whole grains into your daily consumption and will be well worth it later in life. Just like any other aspect of your life; if you put the work in today, you will reap the benefits later; in hopes of a well sculpted, healthy body that is disease free for the better part of life. A healthy grain list is accumulated in the (Appendix, whole grain list, page 94). The dairy world has proven its weight in gold to date! Dairy has a long standing track record of many body building positives and should be a part of your daily life. That being said, let's ensure that you are working with the right dairy; meaning the lowest fat- now termed fat free or skim. You should attempt to have at least a good three servings per day most days if you can. So, why consume dairy products? What can they do for me? Dairy foods provide several important nutrients, including protein, B vitamins and vitamin D, and are considered major sources of calcium in the diet. Eating several servings of dairy foods throughout each day can help prevent calcium deficiency. Calcium deficiency can lead to the breakdown and loss of bone tissue and increase the risk of developing the bone-weakening disease osteoporosis later in life; yes, men can have osteoporosis too! Protein in dairy is one of the highest biological proteins we have in our food supply; an important tool in developing muscle growth and maintenance. Let me also take the time to introduce the whey protein shake. This can be readily used as a snack or meal on the go, and comparably on most occasions can be quite equitable to a dairy serving or two. There is a long list of manufacturers of so called whey protein powder. I would suggest that you seek out a manufacturer that has been on the market for many years and has built a name that symbolizes quality. The B-vitamins from dairy in general help the processes in your body to get or make energy from the food you eat. They also help form red blood cells which transport the oxygen throughout your body. Vitamin D helps your body absorb calcium, which your bones need to grow. In addition, it is proving to be very important in reducing the risk of cardiovascular disease (heart attacks and strokes) when presented in optimal amounts in the blood with focus on higher vitamin D containing foods; supplementing with Vitamin D is still being researched (Brandenburg, 2012, Gouveri, 2012, and Van de Luijtgaarden).

So, what if I do not like dairy or I am lactose intolerant? The good news is that if you do not like dairy in general, you can pick up the nutrients noted above through other food groups in your daily consumption. High biological protein, you can find in any animal flesh, egg, and seafood or soy product. B vitamins you can find in optimal amounts in the grain group (natural and fortified), protein foods noted above and leafy greens. Calcium can be found in green vegetables, and vitamin D in fortified foods such as cereal, and orange juice. In addition, it can be found naturally in oily fish, liver and some mushrooms. Vitamin D may be a warranted supplement if you do not consume any of the above; which would be hopefully highly unlikely. Supplements will be discussed in another chapter, but all proposed supplements should be a conversational piece with your primary care physician before using. If you are lactose intolerant, believe it or not, most of the noted dairy items have a "lactose free" version on the market today! I too am lactose intolerant to a certain extent, as I can consume only hard cheeses; room temperature dairy tends to bother me. Therefore, loving all dairy, I purchase the lactose free versions to assist me in my dairy counts! Now, I am not saying never to consume that banana split or that regular large bowl of Mint Chocolate Chip ice cream. Heck, we all have our downfalls and our weak points in life. I will tell you to severely limit those times. If not, you will be enjoying mid-life with attempting to lose that weight to alleviate the pain in your knee joints, trying to reduce your elevated blood sugar and blood pressure! So, enjoy, but do not regularly indulge; be smart! A list is accumulated in Appendix, Commonly eaten dairy products, page 95.

In all the above food groupings there are some noted serving sizes and recommended number of portions to consume on a daily basis. The serving portions of each group will vary. These are noted in the appropriate appendix.

Fats should be consumed on a limited basis. They should be consumed sparingly simply because of their given calorie content. However, if you are on the leaner side you may want to include a few servings into your daily diet. The best types of fats to consume are unsaturated fats. There are two types, mono and polyunsaturated. These are the fats that assist in fighting disease states such as heart disease. Rich sources of unsaturated fats are nuts, avocados, and unsaturated oils such as olive and canola. The artery clogging, heart disease fats are called saturated fats. These are typically found in animal derived products, more prominent in fatty cuts of meats, and higher percentage of fat dairy products such as whole milk. These too are found in processed foods if animal products were used to develop. Therefore you should do your best to limit these types of fats. Another bad fat is trans-fats. These were typically found only in man-made foods, processed foods. They are weaning their way out of our food due to more restrictions put on by government watchdogs. However, they are still present in the processed foods; thus limit. See Appendix for healthy list of fats, page 97.

How about fluids Joe? I will address this in the beginning but it stands for each decade from here on out. If you plan on being active, as I am preaching, you will require more fluids due to body needs- sweat response, thermal regulation (keeping your body temperature in check), and overall hydration. Fluids also help excrete waste products from the body. Thus adequate hydration is a must. To provide some numbers for you, I would consume at least 75% of your fluids per day from pure old water. I consume tap/city municipal water, but be my guest and consume whatever type you wish as long as it is calorie free. I will only repeat this once in a much later chapter as fluids are very important throughout the lifecycle but grow increasingly important in the latter stages. That said, a standard to aim for each day would be about 8 ounces per waking hour. Yes, you may be going to the bathroom a good bit, this should happen as it would be considered natural. However, remember, with the consumption of all fluids you are performing many important body processes such as providing hydration, helping metabolism, and promoting satiety to suggest a few. All fluids do count, but remember to try to consume at least 75% from water, and yes, carrying around a water bottle with you would assist tremendously as at the very least it will serve as a reminder to drink! See appendix for ACSM fluid replacement recommendations, page 98.

Exercise

Building a foundation for life! If you have not "worked out" regularly in your teens or early 20's now is the time to get moving. This will be imperative for many reasons for an optimal life cycle. First and foremost, it will assist heavily in "keeping lean," second, it will assist with keeping internal stress levels under control (a natural stress reducer), third, it will keep your vanity, for a male in his 20's this cannot be understated of course, and fourth, it will be very personable for you as this will remain your daily devotion to "self!" You will need to learn to carve out this time, early morning, noon or night to continue staying the course over the life cycle as more responsibilities and life in general takes hold. In addition, you will also need to be *creative and flexible* in "getting in" your workouts! This may mean one day you will have to work out at 4 AM, and another on your lunch break or you may have to split it up such as doing your cardiovascular work in the AM and your resistance training in the PM. If you truly dedicate yourself to your foundation work, it will be a no brainer (a part of who you are) later down the road in life. It will be just as a part of your day as taking a shower, as it should be! Remember, you owe it to yourself to take the best possible care of YOUR body!

So, we are going to start with the basics. I will assume we are all beginners here and thus all desire to learn what we can about exercise and how to incorporate it into our daily lives. For the newbie's out there let's start with some basic exercise goals. If this is the first time you have exercised in your life we need to start slow. This will provide us with a working knowledge of the "how" piece of exercise. It is important to first start with ensuring that this is tolerable to your lifestyle and your body. Follow the progression below.

1) Walk 3 days per week for 30 minutes for the first 4 weeks (this can be outside or on a treadmill)

   Keys to success for walking:

   a) Ensure you purchase appropriate footwear (walking, running or cross training sneakers) and comfortable workout clothing.

   b) Purchase a stopwatch- this will be your most precious tool in the long run.

   c) Partner up if you must- only those with the utmost perseverance can do this all alone. That being said, you also *better learn* to do this all on your own as you may sometimes never have a partner and must solely rely on your own fortitude to get through it. I have had well over forty partners to date and have either burned them out, or schedules changed and I had to persevere on my own. Get to the point that you realize that you are in this game of life by yourself and not only will you persevere, but you build that self-confidence!

2) Walk 5-6 days per week for 45-60 minutes for the next 3 weeks. You may add in biking or swimming to this if you like to change up the pace but that would be all for right now. This is a crucial point, as we are building up the frequency piece of exercise during this portion in addition to your exercise tolerance.

3) Now, we are at 6 days per week of exercise; good! To date, you have built up your frequency and exercise tolerance. Let's now build that body's foundation! I want you to start with the basics of building the human body (Appendix- Basic bodybuilding exercises, page 100) for display. I want you to start a rotation of the following for three- 30 minute sessions per week- pushups, sit ups and body weight squats. Simple! I want you to do them in the following sequence:

a) <u>3 days per week</u>
   i) Pushups (as many as you can and yes, you can vary your arm length and feet width if you choose)
   ii) Sit ups (as many as you can)
   iii) Body weight squats (as many as you can)
   iv) 1-2 minute break (use that stopwatch)!
   v) Repeat for 30 minutes.
   vi) 30 minutes of cardiovascular activity- at this point you can still walk, bike or swim. However, if you have access to another piece of equipment such as a rower, elliptical machine or other piece of equipment, you may also incorporate these. This puts us at 60 minutes total at three

days per week.

b) <u>3-4 days per week</u>

    i) Walk, bike, swim or cardiovascular piece of equipment for at least 45 minutes

    ii) We will be doing this for the next 4 weeks!

4) After this four weeks we have really made progress! You should really start to see changes in your body, strength, definition and you clothes may be a tad looser. We will now incorporate a tad more resistance but keeping with the same theme, 3-4 days of weight/cardiovascular exercise, and 3 days of only cardiovascular activity. Do not be concerned of the actual days of the week this falls. Just ensure that first, you get them all in, and second that you try to have a cardiovascular day at all times in between your resistance days. This will give us our basis for a lifelong body and workout that becomes "routine" to us because now it is manageable and can fit into our everyday lives- no matter how stressful they become. At this point, you may want to invest in two things, a gym membership or some decent pieces of home gym equipment. (Appendix- Home Workout Basics, page 102). The recommendations on home equipment will prove its worth over time; especially as both your career and family life may start taking up more time and a gym is not feasible most of the time. Home equipment will be quintessential in the long run. Invest wisely and build your home work out gym piece by piece as it does not have to be a large assortment, just enough to get the job done!

We will be breaking this down as such, sweet and simple. Before we start, we must understand some basic bodybuilding terms. These terms will all be terms to live by and to use in your everyday "workout" vocabulary!

- *Set*- A set is a collection of repetitions that culminates in the muscle reaching muscular failure (Rivera, 2005). Muscular failure is the point, due to a buildup of lactic acid in the muscle, it becomes impossible to perform another repetition with good form.

- *Repetition*- The amount of times that you perform an exercise. For instance, pretend that you are performing a bench press. You pick up the bar; you lower it, pause and lift it up. That action of executing the movement for one time counts for 1 repetition. If you perform that same movement a second time, then that is your second repetition, and so on.

- *Rest interval*- The amount of time that a person rests in between sets. For instance, a rest interval of 60 seconds means that after you finish your first set, you will remain idle for 60 seconds before going on to the next set.

- *Superset*- A superset is a combination of one exercise performed right after the other with no rest in between. There are two ways to implement a superset. The first way is to do two exercises for the same muscle group at once; like doing dumbbell curls immediately followed by concentration curls. The drawback to this technique is that you will not be as strong as you usually are on the second exercise. The second and best way to superset is by pairing exercises of opposing muscle groups or different muscle movements such as Back and Chest, Thighs and Hamstrings, Biceps and Triceps, Shoulders and Calves, Upper Abs and Lower Abs. When pairing antagonistic exercises, there is no drop of strength whatsoever once your cardiovascular system is well conditioned.

- *Drop set*- Drop sets are exactly what they sound like. You start at one weight then drop to a lesser weight and continue to exercise then drop the weight even lower and finish the exercise to "exhaustion."
- *Barbell*- a bar with adjustable weighted disks attached to each end that is used for exercise and in weight lifting.
- *Dumbbell*- A short-handled barbell 10-12 inches long that can be carried in one hand. Dumbbells allow for flexibility in the execution of a movement and for full range of motion.

1. ***Day 1***- Upper body (Chest, Back, Shoulders, and Abdominals) - 40-45 minutes

   1) **Chest**

      a) Pick one of the following:

         i) Incline bench press (barbell or dumbbell)

         ii) Flat bench press (barbell or dumbbell)

      b) Pick one of the following:

         i) Incline bench dumbbell flye

         ii) Flat bench dumbbell flye

      c) Perform 1 warm up set of each (pick a weight that you can do for at least 12-15 repetitions)

      d) Perform working sets (sets to be included and count after the warm up set) of the following repetition range-12, 10, 6-8, 6-8. Thus, only four working sets; noting after each set, picking an abdominal exercise to complete during your rest interval of 1 to $1^{1/2}$ minutes ONLY. After the first exercise, move on to the next with abdominal exercises in the rest interval phase. This is my coined term "*transitioning workout*." You will create a very high calorie burn during this type of workout; thus providing you with the most bang for your buck. As you will find that this type of workout may be more conducive to your lifestyle as it will get busier as you age and this type of training program will be your survival tool. This provides you with the ability to "know" that you will be always able to get in your workouts when you do have time restraints.

2) **Back**
   a) Pick one of the following:
      i) Lat pulldown, reverse pulldown or other varying grips, pull ups, dumbbell row.
   b) Pick one of the following:
      i) Low back extension, hyperextension bench, physio ball low back extension
   c) Perform 1 warm up set of each (pick a weight that you can do for at least 12-15 repetitions)
   d) Perform working sets (sets to be included and count after the warm up set) of the following repetition range- 12,

10, 6-8, 6-8. Thus, only four working sets; noting after each set, picking a different abdominal exercise to complete during your rest interval of 1 to $1^{1/2}$ minutes ONLY. After the first exercise, move on to the next with abdominal exercises in the rest interval phase.

3) **Shoulders**

   a) Pick one of the following

      i) Shoulder dumbbell, barbell or machine press

   b) Pick one of the following:

      i) Dumbbell, barbell or machine shrugs

   c) Perform 1 warm up set of each (pick a weight that you can do for at least 12-15 repetitions)

   d) Perform working sets (sets to be included and count after the warm up set) of the following repetition range- 12, 10, 6-8, 6-8. Thus, only four working sets; noting after each set, picking a different abdominal exercise to complete during your rest interval of 1 to $1^{1/2}$ minutes ONLY. After the first exercise, move on to the next with abdominal exercises in the rest interval phase.

4) **Abdominals**

   a) You want to work on the three areas of your abdominals (lower, mid and side abdominal muscles) with an array of exercises, weighted and non-weighted; rotating days.

   b) During your workout target one exercise of each lower, mid and side abdominal and rotate through your workout. (Appendix- Abdominal exercises, page 103).

5) **Cardiovascular finish**

    a) Finish your workout with 15-20 minutes of "intense" (feel like you are working at a non-conversational pace) cardiovascular exercise.

2. *Day 2*- Cardiovascular day (45-60 minutes-bike, swim or cardiovascular piece of equipment); push yourself!

3. *Day 3*- Lower body/arms -40-45 minutes

1. **Legs**

    a) Pick one of the following

        i) Back, hack, machine, or dumbbell squat (always consult a certified personal trainer for correct form before starting as back injuries are a timely set back)

    b) Pick the following:

        i) Leg press or lunges

    c) Perform 1 warm up set of each (pick a weight that you can do for at least 12-15 repetitions)

    d) Perform working sets (sets to be included and count after the warm up set) of the following repetition range- 12, 10, 6-8, 6-8. Thus, only four working sets; noting after each set, picking a different abdominal exercise to complete during your rest interval of 1 to $1^{1/2}$ minutes ONLY. After the first exercise, move on to the next with abdominal exercises in the rest interval phase.

2. **Arms**

    a) Pick one of the following (these you will work together as a superset, starting with your tricep exercise choice and moving to your bicep exercise choice).

    i)   Tricep extension, overhead extension, dumbbell kickbacks, close grip bench press or dips.

  b) Pick one of the following:

    i)   Dumbbell or barbell curls, ez curl bar or preacher curl

  c) Perform 1 warm up set of each (pick a weight that you can do for at least 12-15 repetitions)

  d) Perform working sets (sets to be included and count after the warm up set) of the following repetition range- 12, 10, 6-8, 6-8. Thus, only four working sets; noting after each set, picking a different abdominal exercise to complete during your rest interval of 1 to $1^{1/2}$ minutes ONLY. After the first exercise, move on to the next with abdominal exercises in the rest interval phase.

4. **_Day 4_**- Cardiovascular day (45-60 minutes-bike, swim or cardiovascular piece of equipment); push yourself!

5. **_Day 5_**- Same as day 1 but pick different exercises- upper body (Chest, Back, Shoulders, and Abdominals) - 40-45 minutes and 15 minute cardiovascular finish.

6. **_Day 6_**- Cardiovascular day (45-60 minutes-bike, swim or cardiovascular piece of equipment); push yourself!

7. **_Day 7_**- IF YOU CAN- Cardiovascular day (45-60 minutes-bike, swim or cardiovascular piece of equipment) or use this day to rest and enjoy another physical activity like a pickup basketball or flag football game or enjoy a bike ride or long walk.

At this point you have surely increased your lean body mass and have decreased your fat mass. Your metabolism should be raised to a good point to where it should be as an active male in his twenty's. You should feel healthy, motivated and invigorated! Do this workout plan for life; for at least 8 weeks. After 8 weeks, assess. Questions to ask yourself as a self-assessment after 8 weeks: Am I where I want to be? Do I feel I can do more? Am I comfortable where I am at with myself, my work, my social life? Is there a balance? Is my dietary plan where it needs to be to reap the true benefits from my workouts? After this assessment, either continue to advance, or if you are comfortable where you are currently at, maintain your efforts. If you were to advance I would consult a personal trainer or a well-known bodybuilding reference book for increase intensity workouts to get you where you want to be. Remember, you are in this race in life by yourself; *you are your only measuring stick*; no one else! Be comfortable in your own skin! An additional note on testing and challenging yourself; ever so often you may choose to test yourself with increased weight to measure your strength such as on a bench press. I am all for this as it is a good measure for you and keeps the fire burning inside to progress. That being said, it should be safely done with someone who will spot you and it should only be done at the very most once every 3-4 weeks, not more often than this. Remember our goal is to stay lean, strong and in the game of life as fit as we can and for the entire life cycle; being able to move a mountain will serve no purpose in our goal. You should add these challenge sets in at every stage of life.

Injuries

Okay, I would be lying if I told you that you will glide through life working out and NOT have any setbacks. The reality of being part of the "being fit," or "working out" class is that you WILL face injuries from time to time. Some will be acute and only happen from time to time, while others will be more chronic and you will be dealing with them for quite possibly the rest of your life. This is where, you, the individual comes into play. Simply because it is up to you and your attitude how you tackle injuries. You must have a "game plan," or "protocol," if it is a chronic injury, of how you will work around these issues. If it is the first time you are experiencing a pain and you can deduce that it is only mild inflammation, then treat with ice, heat and Non-Steroidal Anti-Inflammatory Drugs (NSAIDS), such as Ibuprofen, Naproxen, or Aspirin; until pain alleviates. More research is pointing towards the use of ice, however use what you find the most relief from. Ensure that you review and follow the directions on the NSAIDS very carefully. If this is a first time injury, you may want to consult with your PCP first for a treatment plan. That being said, if this is a more severe injury, such as a sharp pain in your shoulder, knee or hamstring, just to name a few common problematic areas; consult with your PCP. If it is severe, he/she may refer you to a specialist such as an orthopedic surgeon for continuous care.

Now, covering all the above, a dose of reality is to tell you that this will happen again and again as long as you continue to work out. Therefore, try to identify what caused the pull, strain, or pain. What exercises should I modify, or eliminate all together because it will make me more prone to putting me on the sidelines again? Know these exercises and proceed with caution! Modify, modify, modify; that is the key to staying in the workout game. Work around injuries; never stay on the sidelines. What I mean by this, just because you hurt your shoulder does not mean you should ignore working out altogether! Talk with you PCP or specialist and develop a plan of action. For example, work with limited exercises and/ or work on a pain scale, if your PCP or specialist will allow you. For example, he/she may tell you that they will allow you to work up to a 3 or 4 on a pain scale of 10. If you feel you are hovering over a 4, you would back off of the weight or the actual exercise. Likewise, using the shoulder as an example, even if you must remain off the weights for a period of time, this does not mean you must take the time off! You still have legs don't you? Go to the gym and work on leg machines or cardio equipment that does not involve the upper body such as bike or step mill work. The secret to longevity in the workout game is simply consistency and routine! You will overcome this injury sooner or later and you will not have gotten out of the loop and your consistency would have remained constant.

Remember these key points. Always do the following with injuries:

1. Keep your PCP or specialist in the loop to your injury status.

2. Know your treatment protocol- developing one for new injuries and following developed protocols for reoccurring injuries.

3. Stay consistent with your workout efforts- this is the key to a life filled with adversity that you will certainly have! Remember, it will always be how you attack a situation that will determine the outcome. Keep your head high (positive) and keep moving forward.

4. Injuries will happen! I view my injuries as time to take a step back and dial down on my intensity for a while. I view injuries as my body

telling me to slow down a tad. Your muscles have memory. When you get back to your usual routine they will respond thus the hard work gained earlier will not be lost. If you view your injuries in this light, it is nothing but positive!

Rest and Recovery

Let's address this early on in your 20's as just like these other sections, you will need to realize the importance of obtaining optimal rest and recovery from your workouts and life in general. A key phrase I will very often use is *"*sleep cures all.*"* When you think about in a general sense, it is our creator's way of resetting our clock. Sleep is when you and your body rest. However, while you are resting, metabolism is lower and your body's restorative systems such as your immune system is going to work; pulling the night shift if you will. This is the time when your body regulates itself and provides the necessary patch work such as de-stressing and fighting situations such as colds. In fact, for most of the sleep, about 75% of time, is the time when your muscles are relaxed, additional blood supply is provided to the muscle and tissue growth and repair is completed. Additionally, energy is restored and hormones such as growth hormone are released which is dependent for muscular and other systems growth and development (National Sleep Foundation). In the toxic world we live in where a stressful life is the norm, there is almost nothing that rates close to the importance of proper sleep and sleeping patterns. You will find that very closely to nutrition and your workouts that sleep will also be a defining part of your longevity. You must dedicate yourself to have seven to eight hours of sleep per night. This will set your body up for success the next day as you will feel more energized and ready to take the day on. In addition, stress levels and hunger levels will be lower if this optimal level of sleep is obtained (National Sleep Foundation). Just remember that sleep resets your body back to its programmed "defaults," and sleep "cures all!" Listen to your body as you age and become more in tuned to yourself! When you treat your body well, you will be able to pick up on its inherent signs of telling you what it needs. Sleep is the one thing that you must respond to when your body tells you it needs! Later in life sleep may be more challenging to fit in due to more responsibilities, etc. This is why I am describing and pleading that you see its importance now as if you develop these habits now, it will be vitally important to you later in life and you will deem it as a priority; hopefully scheduling it into your life as you progress. In short, it will help you achieve all of your physical goals!

Weight Loss

If you are like most of us and want to drop a few pounds and you tell yourself, I want to get to that point of a healthy "adult given weight," to ensure I can be healthy for my entire life. I am completing the workouts with success, but I need and want to lose a few pounds to visually reap all the benefits I can if I am putting forth all the effort! How should I go about losing weight (unproductive/unhealthy body fat) and keep my gains in muscle (lean body mass)? Remembering one of the first important **BOLD** points I made; *keep it simple*! We are going to easily help you transition this to the diet. Simply put, we need to consume less than we are expending. This is a combination of both through metabolic processes and physical demands on a daily basis. Therefore, let's simply start with decreasing your late PM calories. Our goal will be to lose half to one pound per week. To do this slowly and methodically we will need to decrease 250-500 calories per day. Let's work our way backwards. First, I want you to cut out all after dinner snacking. If you find this a challenge, I want you to substitute one serving only (tennis ball sized) of fruit after dinner for your later snack if you have one or if you feel the absolute need to have one. If you were a dessert eater (I use this term to mean any high calorie snack post-dinner; could be chips, pretzels, ice cream or whatever your vice is that ratchets up your calories), you will be now limited to one serving of fruit, approximately only 80 calories. Do this if you need to every night. One or two nights, try it completely without anything after dinner. A trick that I personally use after dinner, I immediately floss and rinse with mouthwash; this really seems to limit my post-dinner cravings; give it a try!

Second, I want you to take a look at your dinner plate. I want you to think about your dinner plate in the following way; a 70/30 split. Seventy percent of the dinner plate should be lower-starch vegetables (see Appendix, High starch and lower and non-starch vegetable list, page 104) with limited high calorie toppings (use vinegars, vinaigrettes, calorie free spray such as butter spray, or low calorie dressings, etc). The remaining thirty percent should be lean protein (lean chicken, beef, pork, or seafood) that has been baked, broiled, boiled, grilled or sautéed (but not in oil); typically a palm sized version is equal to thirty percent. Do this most days of the week for dinner as this will soon become one of the most weight controlling habits you will need for your entire life!

Now, do this for four weeks. After four weeks, you should conceivably have lost up to four or more pounds. If you find that you have not, we need to review the following:

1. Ask yourself- Have I been loyal to the above? If the answer is NO, review the above and continue until you are successful!
2. If you have been loyal to the above, we need to take a look at the rest of the day.

If you are satisfied with the results to date with your weight loss efforts, keep up with the above plan. If not, and you have been successful with the above but have hit a plateau or you just want to lose a few more pounds, let's continue.

The most important part of the diet is twofold. First, remember that your body is a machine in essence; you need fuel (blood sugar) to run optimally. We need a steady flow of blood sugar to make you move, think, excel, and basically function as a human. That being said, we need to maintain a consistent flow of blood sugar without tapping your excess storage depots (muscle glycogen and liver glycogen). The way we MAINTAIN this is by feeding the body a controlled amount of healthy calories and not an excess of calories that will be stored for later. We do this by consuming more frequent, smaller meals/snacks throughout the day. This is our second most important part of the diet, in that this will assist in making you feel satisfied (satiety).

As we have already touched upon dinner and post-dinner snacking, the rest of the meals/snacks do not deviate too far either. Breakfast should consist of one/two servings of lean protein, one serving of whole grain (Appendix, whole grain list, page 94) and one serving of fruit. A snack, if warranted between breakfast and lunch would consist ideally of a piece of fruit. If you need more to hold you over, I would choose <u>one</u> <u>serving</u> of any type of unsalted or lightly salted nuts. Lunch, would be the same as breakfast. An afternoon snack can be the same as the AM snack, if warranted. I would stick with the above for an additional four weeks or until you have met your goal. There are two more tricks of the trade that will assist you in your efforts as I have used these successfully with all my clients and myself.

1. Consume one, 8 ounce, glass of non-calorie fluid (preferably water) before your first bite of food at any meal or snack. Then consume more calorie free fluid with your meal. Remember the stomach is a muscle too and fluids assist in filling the muscle, in essence will assist in you feeling fuller faster!

2. Immediately following your meal or snack, if time permits and you can, brush your teeth. If you cannot, ensure that you carry around a pack of sugar free gum; pop a piece in directly after your meal. Again, chewing allows your brain to believe you are eating and consuming calories, hence expediting the feeling of fullness.

Primary Care

If you have not been to a Primary Care Physician (PCP) or provider in years or if you do not have a PCP, now is the time to go or locate one and make that appointment. We want to ensure a couple of things at this juncture in our lives. You need to identify with your PCP that your weight is healthy for you at this stage of your life. He/she will likely compare your weight in kilograms (kg) divided by your height in meters squared to assess your body mass index (BMI); however, BMI DOES NOT take into consideration lean body mass; it is only a gross assessment of body weight. Between you and your physician provider you will be able to identify a healthy bodyweight range that you MUST remain within five pounds of for the rest of your life!

- Tests to have completed in your twenties:
  - Routine physical (recommended every 3 years, unless otherwise directed from PCP)
  - Vision-eye exam every two years
  - Hearing- exam every ten years
  - Skin cancer exam- reviewed by PCP at least every 3 years
  - Testicular exam- self exam starting in teen age years- PCP will/should address at physical (http://www.usfhp.net/pdfs/RecScreenin gsMen.pdf)
- Blood pressure checked at least every two years
  - This is my one and only push at this point for the whole book. I am a very religious man. I will not push upon you efforts of my beliefs. That being said, the human body and its longevity, may be based on your blood pressure throughout the life cycle. Some will say this will determine your ultimate life span? If you believe in this, there are several ways to decrease your blood pressure. Some are physical; workout daily, yoga, etc.

Some are mental, candle gazing, meditating and prayer. I pray multiple times each day. Between my physical efforts and my prayer time I believe these efforts are what is truly one of the major reasons why my blood pressure is normal now and why it will remain normal for most if not all of my life. This all being said, find a mental release in life to decrease your blood pressure! Enough said!

- Blood work- as recommended by PCP
- Have your cholesterol checked starting at age 20 if:
  - You use tobacco.
  - You are obese.
  - You have diabetes or high blood pressure.
  - You have a personal history of heart disease or blocked arteries.
  - A man in your family had a heart attack before age 50 or a woman, before age 60

    (http://www.ahrq.gov/ppip/health ymen.htm)
- Always remember to ask for your PCP to mail any laboratory results/other procedure or testing results you have completed and keep track of this information; ideally you may want to data base this information on a computer spreadsheet. In addition, upon leaving your appointment ensure any follow-up appointments you will need. To stay optimally fit for life, you will need the collaboration of both you doing your part and the partnership of your PCP.

<u>Supplementation</u>

Do I need to take any supplements? Let's start with what supplements are for? They are used to "supplement" the diet. If your diet is lacking for any reason a supplement may be warranted. What would include "lacking in diet?" One reason for a supplement may be that someone is completely ignoring an entire food group, such as fruits, vegetables, or dairy. Or, they are picky eaters and only consume certain types of foods such as only highly processed foods. Or, they are a certain type of vegetarian, such as a Vegan; which may require a supplement if the diet itself is not complete. That being said, if you noted the above dietary sections and are following them, then a supplement really is not warranted at this point, unless advised by your PCP. However, I have been taking certain supplements for years and may be a tad biased when it comes to which ones to take. My personal take on certain types, such as a multi-vitamin/mineral supplement, is that it is all about complete coverage of the diet. It appears that this theory may hold water, and only cost pennies on the dollar. A study suggests that a multivitamin, with recommended dosages, not super dosages, of vitamins taken for a long period of time, may reduce the overall risk of cancer in males (Gaziano, J.M., Sesso, H.D., et al. (2012)). Knowing what I know now and looking back to the decade when I was in my twenty's, I would certainly take the following supplements at this stage of life:

1. Multivitamin- a generic is fine but ensures that it only contains up to the RDA amounts; NOT super dosages!
2. Fish Oil- shown to improve blood flow, decrease vascular damage,

(Xin, W., Wei, W., and Li, X. (2012), may play important roles in prevention and treatment of obesity, metabolic syndrome and cardiovascular disease (Ma Y, Lindsey ML, Halade GV.(2012), decrease risk of type two diabetes (Brostow, D.P., Odegaard, A.O., Koh, W.P. et al (2011)), and lower inflammation, (Kiecolt-Glaser JK, et al, 2012). Fish oil is also being researched in areas for its possible effects on depression, kidney disease, and a host of cancers.

3. Calcium and Vitamin D (often sold together in supplement formulas) – can improve bone status when not adequately present in the diet (Morris, H.A., O'Loughlin, P.D., and Anderson, P.H. (2010)), and decreased risk of cardiovascular disease (CVD), (Sun, Q., Shi, L, Rimm, E.B, et al (2011)).

4. To ensure that you are on the same page of research, provide your supplement list to your PCP and discuss with him/her your daily regimen.

Men in their 30s- Moving forward!

The 30's will be a time when you are starting to come into your own! You are following progressive steps in your chosen career. You may or may not have a wife or family. At this point in your life it is critical that you have maintained your "*self-time*." I have witnessed this all too often when I entered my 30's. I had a lot of close friends and acquaintances literally age ten years ahead of me during these years. This was all simply due to not taking and applying what you had read from the decade before! If they had devoted self-time, they either chose to use this time for something else constructive or they supplemented with something unhealthy such as television time. These friends and acquaintances stopped taking care of themselves both physically and nutritionally. Therefore, I have witnessed them gain unhealthy body weight, met with diagnosed hypertension, hypercholesterolemia, type 2 diabetes, knee pain which may lead to knee replacements, and lower back problems, amongst a host of other health issues. Why do they have all of these issues? Why did they do this to themselves? These issues were simply brought about by a substantial increase in weight, but not just weight, unhealthy weight. They have observed a substantial increase in fat mass to lean body mass ratio to be exact. They have simply either increased calories or decreased activity level or both during the past several years and the weight crept on. This is tremendously dangerous as with most of the above diseases; heart disease is looming and cancers may not be too far behind. Once you do receive a diagnosis of a disease such as type 2 diabetes, you will always have this medical label on you and your health insurance no matter what you do. Do not be in this group, especially with the preventable diseases that plague advanced societies such as ours!

<u>Nutrition</u>

Dietary consumption should not deviate too much in your 30's from your 20's. The key still is to consume from the earth with focus on high fiber, high antioxidant foods with peppered in lean protein and dairy on a daily basis. Of concern in this decade of life is the afore noted weight gain. If you have gained a few pounds over the past few years and have not taken any action, think about doing it now! If you are on target and have adhered, move on to the next section, exercise!

<u>Tips to assist in removing some of the added weight</u> with the diet:

1. Review the weight loss section noted in the 20's and implement what is needed.

2. Really look at your current dietary intake. What has changed? What are your dietary triggers? Are you eating out too much? Are you aggressively snacking due to stress/anxiety/depression? We often find comfort in our foods and our food environment. Therefore if you have a certain "life" trigger, this needs to be addressed now as it will certainly start to embed into your daily life until it is truly a part of you. This is where you need to take a look at your life. Do I need help with life struggles? Do I need some type of counseling? If finding comfort in unhealthy foods for life issues it may be wise to address it now before it is too late and your health is truly affected with a life time disease. Seek help if need be.

a. Negative dietary triggers can be dealt with if you have the willpower or the social support. Once realized that you do have a trigger due to a life event(s) and it is being addressed, you must now deal with the dietary component of it. How? I would suggest you not change the reaction to the life event, for example, eating at the point of the trigger, but work with the trigger. I am saying change your response to the trigger. Fulfill the trigger with a healthier option. If your trigger is to aim towards something sweet, try taking apples with cinnamon and stevia and mixing and keeping on hand. If you have a salt trigger, address this with some celery sticks and mustard for that salty crunch. Learn how to deal with your trigger. Look, life will continue to throw us all curve balls; that is a fact! The way we respond to the event is the difference between overcoming the event or being swallowed by the event! Be proactive and test your trigger foods, thus setting yourself up for success. Do not be reactive and try to deal with it after it happens. Practicing these dietary triggers before they happen will hopefully instill that instinctive reaction to your trigger in hopes of creating a caloric friendly environment for you to lose that excess weight.

3. If you truly feel that you are completely out of control, seek the guidance of a Registered Dietitian to assist you at this time. He/she can provide you with the reinforcement tools that you

need to get back on track.

Remember, it is imperative that once you get back on track that you keep your calories under control and you eat the recommended amounts of vegetables and fruits per day. This will provide you with a solid foundation for your later years. Time well spent now in addressing the wrong turns will certainly pay dividends later.

Exercise

If you established a routine in your 20's and it has worked thus far, continue your efforts. There is absolutely no reason that you should/have to change your exercise routine. To assist in increasing calories burned and offsetting any potential weight gain, ensure that you are at the very least keeping these useful daily extra steps in your repertoire:

- Take "desk breaks," if you have a mainly sedentary position at work. At least once every hour, peruse the halls and get some water or go to the bathroom or chat with a co-worker for at least ten minutes.
- Stand at work- yes, standing will help you burn more calories and break the complacency of just sitting all day. Find a way to work on your computer when you are standing- when I am in the office I do this many times each day.
- Do some office stretching- examples are easy to find on the internet.
- Take a jump rope to work!
- Park your car a long distance from the building; try that walking thing!

- Take the stairs and avoid the temptation of the elevator.
- Plan field days at work if you can; little trips, such as walking to the post-office or to get some coffee.
- Take that walk after or before lunch!
- If your position at work now or has always required travel or you travel leisurely ensure that you take the basics with you even if you stay at locations where they have a top of the line gym or workout center as you never can tell what will happen and you will always be prepared.
- Good pair of running sneakers
- Breathable workout/running socks
- Loose fitting workout outfits
- Resistance tubes- I usually travel with two- one medium level and one hard level resistance
- Stop watch
- Music- if you need

You can essentially get the same workouts in with a little creativity even when you do not have access to all the gym equipment. Remember, the most important part of each exercise routine is always the same. First, you get it in, and second, that you keep the intensity. If you live with these two notions each workout will prove to be the best that it can be and you will feel that you did your best under any circumstance. See Appendix, Resistance tube exercises, page 106, for exercises that can be used either for travel or a change at home. This may be the time to take a look at the time in which you train if you are having an issue with getting your training time in due to work or family obligations.

Remember, no one said," thou must work out after work!" If you truly dedicate yourself to "your" life you will find a time that is suitable to your schedule. I currently workout at 3:30 in the morning, this is due to my work schedule and current living conditions. It proves to be good for me as I am able to take on all the stressors of the work day, can dedicate my time to extra hours at work if I must, and I am not "sweating" having to get out of work on time to ensure I get to the gym. In addition, this way works for me as I rarely miss any dedicated time to myself; as issues in life tend to evolve once the sun comes up and rarely before! This is just a note if this is a current issue for you, take a firm look at before work, or at lunch versus afterwards.

Injuries

By now these injuries will mostly be of the reoccurring type. You should have established injury protocols that you now follow religiously. You should also be headstrong and viewing these injury "timeouts" as times to re-evaluate your efforts and slow down on the workout accelerator. Give your body time to heal, but DO NOT get out of the game; as noted in the previous chapter, you must stay in the game! Again, if you experience a new injury, see your PCP and discuss a planned attack. This may include seeing a specialist or just discussing a treatment protocol with your PCP that you should follow and follow-up with him/her if need be. Most PCPs or specialist will want to see you in 4-6 weeks to assess the progress. Keep these appointments, as again it is vital to keep the rapport with YOUR medical team.

Rest and Recovery

By now, you likely have developed hopefully strong sleeping patterns and are thriving on the seven to eight hours each night. You are realizing sleep's importance in recovery from your stressful days, workouts, and injuries; noting to yourself that sleep accelerates the positives of all the body's systems. I will not reiterate from the previous chapter, however, this decade I know is when things start to become stressful with family and work obligations. All I can suggest is keep focused on you as a whole person and try to do your best to ensure that you get your rest when you can to help in weathering the events of life. It will deem vital in the later years!

Primary Care

At this point in your life you should have an established rapport with your PCP. Your physicals and other frequent health screenings and tests should be routine in your health prevention repertoire.

However, if you have fallen off the prevention wagon and have not seen your PCP for some time or you just happen to pick up this book in your thirties, now is the time for action! Many of the potential killers both slow, such as some cancers and some fast, such as sudden cardiac death, can be prevented if detected early enough. Most of us are not physicians so this requires that we contact someone who is and make that appointment. Most males, let's face it, are AFRAID! We are afraid to find out that something is wrong with us; it is often the worse news; negative health news! We often wake up in the morning and if we can breathe without an issue, like chest pain, we assume we are in great health. Well my soon to be middle-aged friend, this may or may not be true. The following tests will prove you right or wrong. Make that appointment and put your worries and possible stubbornness aside and take care of yourself starting NOW!

Tests to have completed in your thirties:

- Routine physical (recommended every 3 years, unless otherwise directed from PCP)
- Vision-eye exam every two years
- Hearing- exam every ten years
- Skin cancer exam- reviewed by PCP at least every 3 years- Ensure that your PCP takes a look at your entire body, especially areas you cannot see on a regular basis such as your back. If there is anything questionable, mole or spot, see if you can schedule an appointment with a Dermatologist to review. Take a picture of the mole or spot with your cell phone and monitor it on a regular basis.
- Testicular exam- self exam starting in teen age years- PCP will/should address at physical (http://www.usfhp.net/pdfs/RecScreenin gsMen.pdf)
- Blood pressure checked at least every two years
- Blood work- as recommended by PCP
  - Add/ask your PCP about drawing blood work on your hormonal pool to primarily check your testosterone levels at this point. They tend to dip in your thirties and into your forties and you and your PCP can discuss appropriate medication if warranted and agreed upon.

Have your cholesterol checked starting at age 20 if:

- You use tobacco.
- You are obese.
- You have diabetes or high blood pressure.
- You have a personal history of heart disease or blocked arteries.
- A man in your family had a heart attack before age 50 or a woman, before age 60 (http://www.ahrq.gov/ppip/health ymen.htm)
  - Not to reiterate from the prior chapter, but will do since I know I am dealing with men in this book and we like and sometimes need reiteration! Always remember to ask for your PCP to mail any laboratory results/other procedure or testing results you have completed and keep track of this information; remember that you may want to enter this on a computer spreadsheet and keep in a health folder. In addition, upon leaving your appointment ensure any follow-up appointments you will need are scheduled. To stay optimally fit for life, you will need the collaboration of both you doing your part and the partnership of your PCP.

This is also the time to establish a relationship if you have a chronic condition that your PCP feels is better to be managed by a specialist, such as a Cardiologist or Endocrinologist. They too need to be in your health prevention loop; keeping these appointments and making them as important as your workouts and dietary efforts will prove vital as life moves forward.

Supplementation

All of the supplements you are taking or are thinking about taking for whatever reason should be discussed with your physician. You should have an established rapport with your physician provider thus this may not require a visit. I often call my PCP and leave a voicemail for him with a question or comment, in this case a supplement, and he timely contacts me with his opinion. You want this type of working relationship with your PCP. As noted in the prior chapter I would retain the multivitamin, fish oil, calcium and vitamin D. If new research surfaces and has a positive track record about a new supplement or combination thereof and is proven to prevent, assist or relieve some type of ailment or chronic condition run it by your PCP. Be smart, if you have the time, diligently conduct your own research, check documented research articles- you can use websites such as http://www.ncbi.nlm.nih.gov/pubmed.

Men in their 40s- Times are getting serious!

So we are in the decade of responsibility. This may be different on many levels for each man whether it is coming from the angle of family growth, job growth, or more responsibilities from other outside activities from developed opportunities. This is the time in your life where the "rubber meets the road" in the most true sense. I want you to take a look around at your friends in the same age group. Have they taken care of themselves to date? Are most of them carrying around at least 10-20 pounds more weight than they should? I am betting that if they do see their PCP that a handful or even all have high blood pressure, or type II diabetes or are at least on the pathway of having one or the other, or both. This is the testament decade. Have you been truly able to develop into your daily life those "standards of care" for self that were heavily noted in the aforementioned chapters? Have you dedicated that time for you; that *self-time*? Have you made it important to you to carve out this time on a daily basis? Is it standardized in your planner or embedded in your daily planning? If it is not by now, why not? Is it just a time issue? Is it an over commitment issue? Is it laziness? These are questions that you need to reflect on now if you are not taking care of yourself. Simply put, if you have not retained what you have done prior for yourself, or have not started; when are you going to get started? When is your life going to be valuable to you? Typically life gets harder as we move forth, not easier. Responsibilities will become more complex and more important than ever. If you are not already positioning yourself for success it will be hard to integrate something new into your life. Now, this all being said, I have witnessed men in their 40's visit the emergency room for their first "chest pressure" event. Do not be one of them. The day starts now! If you have always taken care of yourself, congratulations and keep on progressing. If you have but stopped for some reason, take a step back and reassess. Reach out to focus on what works or what had worked for you. Take a step back and truly realize that without your health you will not be able to help others! If you have not taken care of yourself at all, now is "THE" time to start as the life cycle time clock is ticking!

Nutrition

There is not much that has changed. I am approaching this section as if you have followed the above and are progressing. Nutrition consumption from the 3rd decade to now will not change too much. The one concern I have for every man is simply the over committed man. Too many responsibilities often lead to too many days and nights of over consuming too many calories. Therefore, my lead into this chapter for nutrition will solely focus on keeping calories under control.

I want you to take a brief look into your dietary history at the moment over the past year or so. I want you to identify your "trigger" foods. What are your go to foods when you are short on time, over stressed, bored, etc? How often have these foods foiled your plans to get where you physically want to be? If your answer is more than once than keep reading! We have to establish a simple foundation here when it comes to these types of "trigger" foods which are often calorically laden. How do we do this? Well, in my life, I simply do not buy these foods! This does take some extreme will power, but I understand that you may have a wife, and/or children and they do not want to join your "healthy" crusade or they do but just not every day- though it would truly not be a bad idea. Simply put the more the merrier as it would be more of a simplified lifestyle if you can have a group moving forth and tackling an issue versus just one man! We know in life through research that the environment is everything. A supportive environment, in this case, not having the food within grabbing distance of the man, would assist in providing a positive outcome; keeping the waist line in check! This has proven to be the most effective approach to these types of "trigger" foods. That being said, there are some happy mediums. However, these are less recommended simply because they take will power and discipline. If you have a hard time with discipline it is best to keep these foods completely out of sight for the time being until discipline can be developed and sustained. You can develop a reward system with yourself. I completely understand that this is a beautiful life. Part of this life is tasting all that it has to offer; I am on board with this concept as I too treat myself for being very good! So, to look at an example, let's say your "trigger" food is pizza. Typically you would likely order this for takeout/delivery or at a restaurant. However for the sake of the example let's say you have it readily available on speed dial. I am not against pizza; especially coming from a hearty appetized southern Italian family heritage. That being said, I have common sense. Too much of a rich food source (excess calories) will devoid my hard efforts to keep me fit and will lend to grossly develop the southern Italian family heritage genes; short and stout! Therefore, I would set something up like the following. I would say to myself that if I am good for two weeks, meaning I completed all my workouts and have kept within reasonable limits of my dietary plan, I can have a personal sized pizza. On this pizza however, I will keep to items that are lower in calories. When I order I would tell them to go light on the cheese, add all types of vegetables or even deli ham or sardines, an acquired taste. See, to me this is what is called a compromise. I love pizza and it is one of my own "trigger" foods. I only have pizza once or twice a year. I cannot have it around, and only order with friends or family who know me and know how I treat my body; therefore when I do order, they know it is a very special time. I am okay with that as this is my reward system. Remember, life is short and should be sweet! Taste all, and leave nothing behind, but be reasonable. If you have "issues," with your "trigger" foods, do not buy them. If you can come to a decent compromise and have the will power to do so, then go ahead. Remember, it is your body and only you, and of course your genetics, have the power!

If weight loss is still a primary issue for you, please refer to the former chapters on how to assist.

<u>Exercise</u>

This is time to take a step back and assess your workouts. Ask the following questions.

1. Have my workouts been consistent?
2. Have I been giving my all during the workouts?
3. Am I excited to workout?
4. Am I setting myself up to receive the benefits from my workouts?

Let's be completely honest. If you have been on the straight and narrow and everything is working out with all the above questions, then stick with it! I will tackle each of the questions for those that have been having issues with their workouts. Consistency is the key to keeping yourself physically and mentally engaged in your health for the life cycle. I had alluded to this more than once prior. Men who are "exercisers" for life will lead happier and hopefully less diseased lives than those who are not as devout. If you are having issues with consistency, you must ask yourself why? Again, going back to the prior chapters; is it because you now have a love affair with your couch? Have you not been able to carve out the time in your schedule? Have you lost your "mojo?" If you need this consistency back maybe the following tips will help.

1. Identify a time slot that is a good time for you to workout- Make sure to keep the excuses at the door. Yes, you may have to wake up an hour earlier or shift your schedule. However, if your health is a priority to you, then you will. If it is not, then you can continue to complain and things will only get worse, including your physical and mental health. Keep this time slot dedicated to you! This means short of a death or family emergency this is your time!

2. Find some motivation. Look, we all have days that we go through the motions. However, this should not be every day. Sometimes workouts can become stale. That being said, find something that motivates you. The workouts provided were developed for men who want the most bang for their buck and can focus within themselves to make the best of it. The aforementioned workout is not the only one out there. Find one

that works for you! Maybe increasing the intensity by cutting down on your rest time in between sets? Maybe trying new exercises to rotate in with your workouts? Maybe change around your home gym? Maybe change the music or upload more music? Maybe substitute a mixed martial arts class for a cardiovascular workout session? Whatever you need to motivate you, find that one thing that you need.

3. <u>How to find my mojo?</u> I admit, I have lost my mojo from time to time in my life. However, I always related this to things that were going on outside of my workout life. Things such as relationship issues, work stress, etc. Then I remember that my workouts were one of things that were my standards, my saving grace, my sanctity; simply because that was the time I could dedicate to myself and relieve those outside stressors. This type of thinking often brought me back into my mojo. However, if you still cannot find it, you may want to take a look at what is going on outside of your workout life; understanding that you may have to address those issues first if you are to continue to thrive in other areas of your life. Remember, that your workouts are FOR you to enable yourself to tackle life and all its stressors. Your workouts are there to enable you to move forth and keep a lower stress perspective even in life's most difficult moments.

4. <u>Am I giving 100% in my workouts?</u> If to date you have had limited success in your physical and mental health, you may want to review your workouts. Ask yourself; have I been giving them their due effort? Have I been going into them wishing they

were over with? Have I been destroying my workouts with my poor dietary consumption? Remember this; you will only get out what you put in. This applies to not only your workouts and dietary consumption but yes, even in life as a whole. Consistent workouts are the absolute key to keeping active throughout life and giving yourself the ability to stroll into your next decade of life with the fairest chance of successful health. Just remember, one key phrase that I will continue to revisit, is to remember that *__metabolism is everything__. Consistent workout efforts allow you to retain your lean body mass and retain or decrease fat mass. Keep progressing!

Rest and Recovery

Sleeping patterns should now be established. You are either proving to yourself that you have found your sleeping pattern and are accelerating in all aspects of your whole self, or you are completely upside down with your sleeping habits. You will easily be able to see its trail. If you are super-stressed, gaining weight, not recovering from sickness or injuries from your workouts; start by examining your sleep habits and sleep schedule. I would think if all the above is running smoothly you are on track. If you have issues with sleeping and cannot figure out why, I implore you to discuss this with your primary care physician. I am not saying that this could be something more serious; I am just saying that we need to find out why and have a plan of attack and resolution.

Injuries

Unfortunately injuries will likely continue to rear their ugly head. Yes, this may provide a minor setback to your physical and mental health efforts. However, do not despair, try to take them in stride. For example when I experience a repeated injury, I fall back on my treatment protocol for each injury. For example, my lower back treatment is as follows:

1. Non Steroid Anti Inflammatory Drugs (NSAIDs) first 48 hours
2. Heating pad first and second days at work during the day and ice with pressure in the evenings

This is my treatment protocol that I found works for my lower back, by day three pain is typically about 3/10 and dissipates from there. By dealing with my treatment protocols as such it also provides me with a mental lift. I tell myself, that I have been here before and I have always bounced back. Listen to your body, and follow your designed treatment protocol and you will be fine; strong mentality still in check! I want you to also learn from this experience; listen to your body. During this time, I will still workout; however, I modify my workouts. I tell myself that this is good recovery for my body. Remember we just discussed consistency above! Only go to the side line, taking time off from workouts, if it is a severe or new injury and you absolutely cannot work out! Otherwise, find a comparable workout that you can do. Also remember, if it is a new injury and concerns you, seek your PCP or orthopedic for diagnosis and/or treatment. Do NOT exercise in pain. If this is a reoccurring injury and it hangs around much longer than usual, be sure to seek an appointment with your PCP or orthopedic.

Primary Care

Okay fellas let's review our checklist.

1. Have established annual visits or very close to annual visits for physicals with our PCP- check

2. Have established a good, trusting rapport with our PCP- check

3. Have received the care and have followed the screening tests mentioned in the decade of the thirties- check

Have recorded our testing results such as noted earlier in a simple spreadsheet to ensure that we are taking control of our own health care- check

To re-emphasize the recommendations, added screenings in

BOLD:

- Routine physical (recommended every 3 years, unless otherwise directed from PCP)-ask your PCP- I see mine annual!

- Vision-eye exam every two years

- Hearing- exam every ten years

- Skin cancer exam- reviewed by PCP at least every 3 years- Review note made in the 30s for care.

- Testicular exam- self exam starting in teen age years- PCP will/should address at physical (http://www.usfhp.net/pdfs/RecScreenin gsMen.pdf)

- Blood pressure checked at least every two years

- Blood work- as recommended by PCP

    o   Add/ask your PCP about drawing blood work on your hormonal pool to primarily check your testosterone levels at this point. They tend to dip in your thirties and into your forties and you and your PCP can discuss appropriate medication supplements if warranted and agreed upon.

- Have your cholesterol checked starting at age 20 if:
  o You use tobacco.
  o You are obese.
  o You have diabetes or high blood pressure.
  o You have a personal history of heart disease or blocked arteries.
  o A man in your family had a heart attack before age 50 or a woman, before age 60

(http://www.ahrq.gov/ppip/health ymen.htm)

- **Prostate exam**- some PCPs will advise starting in your 40s, others may wait until your 50s. Have this discussion with your PCP. So, be certain that you recognize the importance in these screenings. Remember that the odds are much better when you prevent a condition from happening. However, if you do have one and it is diagnosed early, the outcome is typically much more positive. Simply put, ensure that you follow the recommendations!

Supplementation

Starting off with the most important piece of this section; all of the supplements you are taking or are thinking about taking for whatever reason should be discussed with your physician. These are only supplements, meaning supplemented to the diet. They are not prescription medications. Follow your prescribed medication regiment from your PCP. As of current research, as I write this section in 2016, I would retain the multivitamin, fish oil, calcium and vitamin D. If new research surfaces and has a positive track record about a new supplement or combination thereof and is proven to prevent, assist or relieve some type of ailment or chronic condition run it by your PCP. Be smart, if you have the time diligently conduct your own research, check documented research articles- you can use websites such as http://www.ncbi.nlm.nih.gov/pubmed.

Men in their 50s- The new 40s!

The nice thing about taking care of yourself over the life cycle is that you always tend to look much younger than you actually are! I simply believe that if you do take control of your health this is part of the reward. The effects are more than just the appearance on the outside; the insides could also be aging much slower! I believe that is what we are all after, to look, and to feel much younger and to stay around as long as we can in optimal health. However as nice as all the above sounds we still need to focus on maintaining all of our efforts. It is inevitable, even those who have been working very hard to seek optimal health since their early years will unfortunately have to dial it back a tad in maybe the workout spectrum. That said, don't do it just because you are now in your 50's! This is a time in your life where you will likely still have another 15-20 years left in your chosen career. If you are like me, and a lot of men that maintain their health, it helps tremendously to stay physically AND mentally engaged every day. For a lot of us, staying challenged through daily engagements and the economy, may implore us to keep on working for as long as we can. There has been research that viewed longevity in countries where folks work well into their 90s and still live a super vibrant life, contribute to society, and have phenomenal health. Not to say that you may want to work into your 90s but keeping completely engaged on all fronts appears to be the secret to hanging around as long as you can.

Nutrition

Our focus, not to overshadow the excess calories and my always dreaded fear of severe weight gain, will be on ensuring that we are fueling the body with the needed levels of consumed antioxidants. We need to ensure that the immune system is still on the front burner of our health. This will be my reoccurring theme for nutrition throughout the rest of the book as we approach those wonderful golden years. Yes, antioxidants were very important from day one. They could have been obtained simply by ensuring first that you consume the recommended amount of vegetables, fruits, and whole grains each day AND that you vary the types consumed. This would ensure a wide and diverse amount anti-inflammatory fighting nutrients. I said consumed for a reason. We do not want to "pop" a pill for these. If there is one thing that we have come to realize through research, is that the whole food is always better than the one single isolated nutrient, micro nutrient, and vitamin or mineral. To revisit, antioxidants neutralize "free radicals" in your blood which are caused by stress. This stress can be brought on by certain inflammatory diseases. Therefore it is vital to have antioxidants ready to fight in your favor and neutralize or kill the stress. On another level, if you do not have sufficient amounts of antioxidants on a regular basis, the stress may win out; thus an inflammatory disease may begin to flourish. So, how do/should men go about this? It is truly not too hard if you ensure the following and if you are already consuming the recommended amounts of.

1. Ensure that you are consuming at least 1-2 servings of vegetable and fruit per meal and maybe snack; if you can, vary your choices when possible.
2. Ensure that you are tackling grains at least 1-2 times per day.

Again, following the recommendations, as grains will have more calories than vegetable or fruit.

Tricks of the trade too can add antioxidants into your body. If you feel hungry, grab a piece of fruit. Or even if you are trying to cut back on your calories, as you may have gained a few pounds, consume a tennis ball shaped piece of fruit right before your meal with an 8 oz glass of water. This will not only ensure another dose of antioxidant but also help start providing you with a feeling of satiety, which will hopefully offset the any potential overconsumption of calories in a meal.

As I have grown in my profession, nutrition and longevity, I have always highlighted the realm of antioxidants from vegetables, fruits and whole grains as being certainly the center piece to everyone's diet. In fact, I typically only sprinkle in some lean protein choices at each meal to provide me with my ideal dietary plan; to date, it has fared me well. In regards to adding protein to antioxidants, I mentioned before, that I am lactose intolerant. However, thankfully they are now making a slew of lactose free products, so now I have reintroduced them into my regular dietary plan. How much do I love low fat cottage cheese and fruit; a perfect meal!

So, I think you get it by now. Consume your recommended amounts of vegetables, fruits and whole grains. Not only will they fill you with fiber, which will by itself and with other nutrients assist in warding off diseases of the heart, certain cancers and diabetes, but the antioxidants will certainly provide you with the extra layer of defense that we will all need as we age.

Exercise

So this is what I previewed in the opening paragraph. I will note, if there is no need to dial it down, then do not. Keep the train moving forward until you must slow it down for a reason. That being said, if you must dial it down, then be smart about it. Take a step back and remember all the hard work you put into your physical body to date. In addition, remember that it has been a constant in your life to date and your mentality has been sharpened by it. Now, if you must dial the exercise down for whatever reason, then let's address how to do it systematically within the diet. Remember, ***metabolism is everything***. Therefore, if you must decrease the intensity or frequency of your workouts, then you MUST decrease the calories that you will be consuming. The human body will metabolically slow as we age and if you continue to consume the same calories you had previously when you were more active, you will inevitably increase your weight. My fear here is not the 1-2 pounds, but 10-20 pounds you may add. This will open the door to increasing your chances of developing a chronic condition. To battle this, dietary wise, I would simply start with the following and gauge as you go. This is assuming you are not consuming health killers such as snack cakes, cookies, chips, crackers, candy, alcohol (regularly), etc:

1. Decrease one whole grain serving per day.
2. If you are consuming any higher calorie, deemed healthy food, such as nuts; decrease one or two servings.
3. Alcohol- this is the first time and likely last time I will address. These beverages do have certain antioxidant and blood thinning

properties; discuss with your PCP. However, if you are consuming more than one daily, decrease to only one. This should assist in preventing any immediate weight gain when you decrease your workout intensity or frequency. You will have to assess as you go. However, all this being said, I have worked out with some men almost double my age at times and they were able to keep almost tabs with me; I am 41, do the math. So, just because you reach a certain age, this should have no bearing how you approach your workouts. Again, if they are working, keep them moving forward.

Injuries

I do not want to dwell on this anymore than what is needed. However, if this is the reason why you must dial it down; repetitive injuries are occurring too frequently; then be smart. Certainly modify your workouts to address this. If you must, review your workout plan with a professional such as a skilled and certified personal trainer or even physical therapist could assist and shed some light and direction so that your "dialing down" may not have to be as drastic.

Rest and Recovery

Sleep should be consistent at this point in your life; a mainstay. Your developed patterns should be assisting you in all that you are doing mentally and physically each day. Again, I will reiterate from the previous chapter. If you find that you are having difficulty sleeping, falling asleep, or staying asleep, contact your Primary Care Physician; as sleep disorders tend to increase with age.

<u>Primary Care</u>

Fifty years of age seems to be the new threshold for an abundant amount of testing. These new screenings I see as just baselines for you to have for the future. The new screenings/visits will be in **BOLD:**

- **Routine physical** -Annual
- Vision-eye exam every two years
- **Hearing-** exam every three years
- Skin cancer exam- reviewed by PCP at least every 3 years- Review note made in the 30s for care.
- Testicular exam- self exam starting in teen age years- PCP will/should address at physical
  (http://www.usfhp.net/pdfs/RecScreenin gsMen.pdf)
- Blood pressure checked at least every two years. Take advantage of this being taken anywhere you can to be in the "know". Most pharmacies and even grocery stores have self-administered blood pressure stations.
- Blood work- as recommended by PCP
  - o Add/ask your PCP about drawing blood work on your hormonal pool to primarily check your testosterone. They tend to dip in your thirties and into your forties and you and your PCP can discuss appropriate medication supplements if warranted and agreed upon. Have your levels checked at least every other year if okay with your PCP.
- Have your cholesterol checked starting at age 20 if:

- o   You use tobacco.
- o   You are obese.
- o   You have diabetes or high blood pressure.
- o   You have a personal history of heart disease or blocked arteries.
- o   A man in your family had a heart attack before age 50 or a woman, before age 60

    (http://www.ahrq.gov/ppip/health ymen.htm)

- **Prostate exam-**
  - o   **Digital rectal exam-**Annual
  - o   **PSA (blood test)-**Annual
- **Cancer screening-**
  - o   **Fecal occult blood test-** Annual
  - o   **Colonoscopy-** every 10 years; this maybe earlier if you have a positive family history of colon cancer.
  - o   **or Sigmoidoscopy-** every 3-5 years

One thing that is not mentioned and if you can discuss with your PCP provider would be to have a **baseline stress test (walking the treadmill)**; if you have been taking care of yourself, this may be a null issue with your PCP. However, if you had been diagnosed with any cardiovascular risks this may be warranted at this time or even prior. You may also warrant this simply due to your family history. I started my career in cardiac rehabilitation many years ago. I remember having a discussion with one of our highly experienced and very well-known cardio- thoracic surgeons when we were working out at our medical fitness center after work. He told me, as I remember some 15 years later as clear as day, he said. "Joe, if I had it my way, at the age of 50 **EVERYBODY** would have two tests; a treadmill stress test and a chest x-ray. We could view and likely view and treat the most serious killers, heart disease and a host of cancers, if we could do just this." This has been ingrained in my mind ever since and makes very much sense even 15 years later! Therefore I implore you to discuss this option, of having a treadmill stress test, with your PCP; this can certainly SAVE your life!

Supplementation

At this stage of the life I would seriously consider taking your list to your PCP and discuss what you are taking and why. I am all for taking what I noted in the previous chapter for the duration of life. However, you may be facing some other conditions that a certain supplement may be viewed as equivalent or possibly research has shown either better or certainly may complement a medication in taking to control or treat the conditions. Again, ensure to do your homework and research as much as you can.

http://www.ncbi.nlm.nih.gov/pubmed.

Men in their 60s -Approaching those super golden years!

Don't be in a rush!

You are still likely working, but hopefully the end of the work world may be in sight! There is much to consider entering your sixth decade of life when it comes to approaching your health. Not much will change from your fifth decade. If wheel is not broken, don't fix! However, other issues may have risen, even years prior, such as more responsibility such as from family or work related. This again is just a soft reminder that the natural stress reducer is exercise! At times it can be extremely challenging to focus on yourself and your needs especially if you are going through some very trying times such as a sick loved one. I have seen it. That said, taking care of yourself is not to be seen as vein or selfish, it should be seen as the way you collect yourself on a daily basis so that you CAN tackle the other obligations you have as a husband, brother, uncle, grandfather, friend or co-worker that you may face.

Nutrition

This decade will not differ from the 50s. For optimal dietary input I will continue to preach about the importance of consuming an abundance of vegetables and fruit. If there is any time that is crucial to ensuring your adequate amounts of fiber and antioxidants, it is now. Again, these are vital to weight maintenance and fighting diseases that tend to creep up in this decade such as cardiovascular and certain types of cancers. Yes, like you, the cancers really terrify me. That is why you must control what you have control over. Consuming at least 1-2 servings of vegetable and fruit per meal and maybe snack; vary in types when possible. We must also reiterate the importance of consuming the cardiovascular and cancer fighting whole grain. Ensure that you are eating whole grains at least 1-2 times per day.

This is only of the second time that I am addressing fluids.

I am a huge proponent of water consumption, especially for those men that are extremely active. I also understand that water can be a tad boring. Side note, I typically always put lime or lemon juice in my water at home. I am okay with you consuming non-calorie, non-caffeine alternative in place of water from time to time; such as diet tea, non-calorie flavored sweetener packets, flavored water, etc. Yes, I am also okay with the occasional diet soda! I average about 8 ounces of water or non-calorie fluids per hour per day= about 16 waking hours x 8 = 128 ounces per day. This should be a goal for you each and every day, especially if you are remaining highly active. This is important in this decade as it is in the others, especially since you are one of the most active 60some that there are!

Just as a gentle reminder that if for some reason you find that your workout schedule has decreased for whatever reason, be sure to adjust your calorie levels accordingly.

I will not be repeating and wasting your valuable reading time. Therefore, always turn back to the chapter of the 20's decade for basic nutrition information you may be looking for.

Exercise

This is a great time to go back and review the prior decade. The only issue that would potentially come up is dialing the exercise routine down in intensity or frequency for whatever reason. Review the 50s decade if this is or has happened to you to help offset any potential weight gain.

Injuries

As we age this is likely one of the hardest areas to face. The reoccurring injuries are of course treatable, especially since you have had them so many times they almost become routine. With your proven prescription/protocol to treat them, you can surely endure. It is not these injuries that concern us; it is the new injuries we may have in our later years. These must be taken care of appropriately and addressed immediately. For example, if you experience a new injury in this decade it may be wise to immediately contact your PCP or the orthopedic just in case; planning for the worse. At the very least you can get that professional medical information confirming or denying your worse fears such as a long layoff, if it is that severe. If not, you can discuss a plan of treatment and hopefully work around the injury until it does get better. Remember, if it hurts…do not do it! Simple message!

Rest and Recovery

This is again the time to review your sleeping patterns. You may be retired, cutting your hours at work or possibly still working full time. This all being said, your life now could see potential big changes in your sleeping patterns. If having problems, discuss with your doctor as there are many treatments.

Primary Care

Sixty years of age sees us continuing with the now typical 50's decade testing. The new screening screening/visits will be in

BOLD:

- Routine physical -Annual
- Vision-eye exam every two years
- Hearing- exam every three years
- Skin cancer exam- reviewed by PCP at least every 3 years-
  Review note made in the 30s for care.
- Testicular exam- self exam starting in teen age years- PCP
  will/should address at physical
  (http://www.usfhp.net/pdfs/RecScreenin gsMen.pdf)
- Blood pressure checked at least every two years
- **Abdominal Aortic Aneurysm (AAA) -** one time screening for
  men with a history of smoking.
- Blood work- as recommended by PCP
  - Add/ask your PCP about drawing blood work on your
    hormonal pool to primarily check your testosterone
    levels. They tend to dip in your thirties and into your
    forties and you and your PCP can discuss appropriate
    medication supplements if warranted and agreed upon.
    Have your levels checked at least once every other year if
    you can and okay with PCP.
- Have your cholesterol checked starting at age 20 if:
  - You use tobacco.
  - You are obese.
  - You have diabetes or high bloodpressure.
  - You have a personal history of heart disease or blocked
    arteries.
  - A man in your family had a heart attack before age 50 or

a woman, before age 60

(http://www.ahrq.gov/ppip/health ymen.htm)

- Prostate exam-
    - o Digital rectal exam-Annual
    - o PSA (blood test)-Annual
- Cancer screening-
    - o Fecal occult blood test- Annual
    - o Colonoscopy- every 10 years
    - o or Sigmoidoscopy- every 3-5 years

Just as a note, when you visit your PCP for any reason, be sure to ask him/her if you are up to date on all your testing/screenings. In addition, if you are on any medications, please ask your PCP to review them with you as there may be a reason that you can come off a medication or possibly decrease a dosage. If you cannot keep yourself on track, my hopes are that they will! Be diligent as it is your health!

Supplementation

Again, I will defer to the 50s decade and as a reminder, if you want to try a new supplement- discuss it with your PCP first!

<u>Men in their 70s and beyond- The Final Frontier. Maybe</u>
<u>or maybe not!</u>

This is the start of the seventh decade and last decade chapter of this book. I am not saying that time will expire after this decade at all; I am just saying that the breakdown of this decade will not shift too much if you are lucky enough to reach your eighth, ninth, tenth or eleventh decade!

If you are like me, I am always looking forward to these days. These are the days in which I can start looking back and enjoying what I have seen to date and what I am looking forward to seeing. I am optimistically looking forward to today and beyond. I certainly have realized the important role of my nutritional, physical, and mental health has played to date and the balance of life that it allowed me to have. I also realize that what I have put into each of the above is what has gotten me this far in life. I know this is me speaking in the future tense, as again I am 41 years old as I write this book. However, this is how I believe and hopefully will feel!

<u>Nutrition</u>

Nutritional needs will certainly vary by individual. This may be very evident at this stage of life and more prominently during this decade; I will forecast that this will be the more or less "retiring" years for most. Some of you may have kept up the rigorous lifestyle, being very active in your workouts and life in general; whereas some of you may have decreased a good bit. This all being said, your activity level should be dictating your overall body needs and hence nutritional consumption. If you have decreased activity level drastically for whatever reason, you may want to review your nutritional consumption especially if you have seen an increase in weight. Again, review the weight loss section in the 20's decade as this will always be relevant. Likewise, if you have loss too much weight, you will also have to review your nutritional consumption and may have to restore additional calories to your daily diet to achieve the balance you desire. During these decades we need emphasize the following and ensure that you are consuming the adequate amounts as the nutrients found in these groups are extremely important to everyday functioning and overall health; protein, fiber, antioxidants, and hydration. These are not the only areas we must ensure for overall health, but in my eyes they are the foremost important. We must ensure that you are consuming at least a palm sized portion of lean protein at least two to three times per day. This can be and should be in addition to a serving or two of lean dairy. Reviewing the first chapter, will assist in retaining your lean body mass and helping to re- invest in continuing your workouts are successful through recovery.

Fiber and antioxidants are next in line. These come from the favorite vegetable and fruit group, in addition to the whole grains. Ensure that you are getting your recommended servings as this will provide that protective barrier to assist in fighting against cardiovascular disease, other inflammatory diseases and keeping sickness away due to the antioxidants.

Fluid in general is vital in these years. As we age and tend to be less active, which I hope is not happening, we become less likely to consume fluids. It is imperative that you consume fluids not only at meals but also in between meals. Again, water is the best fluid; however, all fluids counts toward hydration status. Pay attention to the weather as well as if you remain active, especially in much warmer climates, you will have to consume that much more fluids to remain hydrated. Dehydration may lead to such issues as increased risk of falls, urinary tract infections, dental disease, bronchopulmonary disorders, kidney stones, cancer, constipation and impaired cognitive function (Coca Cola Company-Beverage Institute for Health and Wellness). A great way to help with the protein, fiber, antioxidants and hydration would be to make your own smoothies or comparable commercial brand to your liking. This may make things more palatable and it is a way to ensure you are getting what you need for your body to maintain its efforts during the life cycle.

Exercise

My hopes are that you are still very active, even as much as the third or fourth decade. I hope to find you still dedicated to your exercise routine even though understandably you have had to tone it down a good bit and you have seen strength and likely endurance decrease; this is okay! That said, just because age is slowly taking its toll on the body does not mean you still cannot excel! I had the opportunity to work with the Maryland Senior Olympics in one of my previous positions; simply amazing. I remember seeing many athletes in their 90's taking part in running events! Take on each day as a day to continually build that body of yours; nourishing it with bodybuilding exercises and cardiovascular input to improve the quality and longevity of your life. You will continue to feel the vigor of life if you continue to follow this track. Do not let age deter you; period!

Injuries

By now you have been working around your long-term injury issues; enough said. My only concerns are the new injuries that may creep up. Again, these are the later stages of life and we need to be aggressive in attending to these new injuries. Therefore, immediately contact your PCP or the orthopedic for any new injuries.

Rest and recovery

Sleeping and workout recovery are vital; if having problems, discuss with your doctor as there are many treatments; you should not suffer.

Primary Care

Seventy plus years of age sees us continuing with the below.

- Routine physical -Annual
- Vision-eye exam every two years
- Hearing- exam every three years
- Skin cancer exam- reviewed by PCP at least every 3 years- Review note made in the 30s for care.
- Testicular exam- self exam starting in teen age years- PCP will/should address at physical
  (http://www.usfhp.net/pdfs/RecScreenin gsMen.pdf)
- Blood pressure checked at least every two years
- Abdominal Aortic Aneurysm (AAA) - one time screening for men with a history of smoking.
- Blood work- as recommended by PCP
  - Add/ask your PCP about drawing blood work on your

hormonal pool to primarily check your testosterone levels at this point. They tend to dip in your thirties and into your forties and you and your PCP can discuss appropriate medication supplements if warranted and agreed upon. Again, have checked regularly.

- Have your cholesterol checked starting at age 20 if:
  - You use tobacco.
  - You are obese.
  - You have diabetes or high blood pressure.
  - You have a personal history of heart disease or blocked arteries.
  - A man in your family had a heart attack before age 50 or a woman, before age 60 (http://www.ahrq.gov/ppip/health ymen.htm)
- Prostate exam-
  - Digital rectal exam-Annual
  - PSA (blood test)-Annual
- Cancer screening-
  - Fecal occult blood test- Annual
  - Colonoscopy- every 10 years
  - or Sigmoidoscopy- every 3-5 years

My hopes are that you only have a PCP. However, more specialists may come into the picture, such as Cardiology or even Oncology. That being said, just ensure that each specialist is in communication with your PCP; you must be your own health care advocate! Be vigilant to ensure that this is taking place.

Supplementation

Again, I will defer to the 50s decade and as a reminder, if you want to try a new supplement- discuss it with your PCP first! Also, if appetite decreases for whatever reason or you find a new dentition issue, it is okay to find and use liquid nutrition. There are plenty of pre-mixed meal replacement or snack formulas on the market, both that you can buy or prepare yourself. Liquid nutrition may be a great way for you to supplement calories thus being able to keep the benefits of your hard work and dedication to your body through the years. If you would want further guidance seek out a local Registered Dietitian for assistance, or once again, ask your PCP.

<u>THE END, not of life, just this short book! So life</u>

<u>goes on!</u>

I hope this book has helped you grasp the basic vital concepts that allowed you to take care of your physical and mental health. To attack and survive this life in today's society it is imperative to take care of all aspects of the human body. This means creating that harmony and balance between life's stressors through engagement of lifelong nourishment of the body. I believe that I have harvested all that I came to know to date through learning from others while testing what has worked for me and not overextending my reaches while knowing my mental limits. The strongest point that I can drive home to you in this closing paragraph is to ensure that you are good to yourself and commit your life to having lifelong "you" time which should be counted as your physical work, your workouts. Problems and issues in life will occur; it is up to you how you attack them! With the balance that you have created you can become a solutions oriented person, as now you have established the tools you need to take on the stressors of this rigorous life.

Best Wishes my friend and may you live life to the fullest in peace and harmony!

Joe

References

Brandenburg, V.M, Vervloet, M.G., and Marx, N. (2012). The role of vitamin D in cardiovascular disease: From present evidence to future perspectives. *Atherosclerosis:* 1- 11.

Brostow, D.P., Odegaard, A.O., Koh, W.P. et al (2011). Omega-3 fatty acids and incident type 2 diabetes: the Singapore Chinese Health Study. *AJCN* ; May 18. 24. Centers for Disease and Control. (February 1, 2013).

NHANES: Healthy Weight, Overweight, and Obesity among U.S.Adults. Retrieved from.
http://www.cdc.gov/nchs/data/nhanes/databriefs/adultweigh t.pdf

Coca Cola Company, Beverage Institute for health and wellness (March 15, 2013) http://beverageinstitute.org/us/article/hydration-for-aging-adults-special-considerations/

Gaziano, J.M., Sesso, H.D., et al. (2012). Multivitamins in the Prevention of Cancer in Men: The Physicians' Health Study II Randomized Controlled Trial. *JAMA:* 1-10. doi:10.1001/jama.2012.14641.

Gouveri, E, Papanas, N. et al (2012). Hypovitaminosis D and peripheral arterial disease: Emerging link beyond cardiovascular risk factors. *Eur J Intern Med:* doi:10.1016/j.ejim.2012.07.001.

Institute of Medicine. Dietary Reference Intakes for Energy, Carbohydrate, Fiber, Fat, Fatty Acids, Cholesterol, Protein, and Amino Acids. 2002. Washington, D.C.: The National Academies Press. Retrieved from http://books.nap.edu/openbook.php?isbn=0309085373

Johnson, I.T. (2004), New approaches to the role of diet in the prevention of cancers of the alimentary tract. *Mutation Research*: 551:9-28.

Kiecolt-Glaser JK, Belury MA, Andridge R, Malarkey WB, Hwang BS, Glaser R. (2012). Omega-3 supplementation lowers inflammation in healthy middle-aged and older adults: A randomized controlled trial. Brain Behav Immun. 2012 May

Ma Y, Lindsey ML, Halade GV.(2012). DHA derivatives of fish oil as dietary supplements: a nutrition-based drug discovery approach for therapies to prevent metabolic cardiotoxicity. *Expert Opin Drug Discov*. Jun 24.

Men: Stay Healthy at Any Age. AHRQ Publication No. 10- IP004-A, September 2010. Agency for Healthcare Research and Quality, Rockville, MD. Retrieved from. http://www.ahrq.gov/ppip/healthymen.htm

Morris, H.A., O'Loughlin, P.D., and Anderson, P.H. (2010) Experimental Evidence for the Effects of Calcium and Vitamin D on Bone: A Review: Nutrients. 2010 September; 2(9): 1026–1035. Published online 2010 September 17. Retrieved from. doi: 10.3390/nu2091026

National Heart Lung and Blood Institute. (February 1, 2013) .What are overweight and obesity. Retrieved from. http://www.nhlbi.nih.gov/health/dci/Diseases/obe/obe_diag nosis.html

National Sleep Foundation. (March 15, 2013). What happens when you sleep. Retrieved from. http://www.sleepfoundation.org/article/how-sleep-works/what-happens-when-you-sleep

Oliveira, F.L.C., Patin, R.V., and Escrivao, M., S., E. (2010). Atherosclerosis prevention and treatment in children and adolescents. *Cardiovasc. Ther;* 8(4), 513-528. Recommended Health Screenings for Men (February, 2010). Retrieved from http://www.usfhp.net/pdfs/RecScreeningsMen.pdf

Rivera, Hugo. (2005). The hardgainers bodybuilding handbook: workouts, nutrition and results. New York: Getfitnow books.

Sun, Q., Shi, L, Rimm, E.B, et al (2011). Vitamin D intake and risk of cardiovascular disease in US men and women. *Am J Clin Nutr.* 2011 August; 94(2): 534–542. Published online 2011 June 8. doi: Retrieved from. 10.3945/ajcn.110.008763

The Bogalusa Heart Study. (October 12, 2012). Retrieved from. http://tulane.edu/som/cardiohealth/index.cfm United States Department of Agriculture. (October 30, 2012). Tips to help you eat whole grains. Retrieved from.

http://www.choosemyplate.gov/food-groups/grains-tips.html

United States Library of Medicine and National Institute of Health search database. Retrieved from.
http://www.ncbi.nlm.nih.gov/pubmed

Van de Luijtgaarden, K.M., Voute, M.T., et al (2012). Vitamin D deficiency may be an independent risk factor for arterial disease. *European Journal of Vascular and Endovascular Surgery*: 44: 301-306.

Worldbank. (October 12, 2012). The average life expectancy for Americans. Retrieved from.
http://data.worldbank.org/indicator/SP.DYN.LE00.MA.IN/countries

Xin, W., Wei, W., and Li, X. (2012). Effect of Fish Oil Supplementation on Fasting Vascular Endothelial Function in Humans: A Meta-Analysis of Randomized Controlled Trials. PloS One; 7(9): e46028. Retrieved from. doi:
10.1371/journal.pone.0046028

Yanovski, J.A., Yanovski, S.Z., Sovik, K.N. et al. (2000). A prospective study on holiday weight gain. *N. Engl J Med*: 342:861

Glossary

A list of terms and phrases used in this book

Prevention- Simply used in this book as stopping something, such as effects of poor health, before it starts.

If you do not have your health, you have nothing! - This about sums it up. If you do not have your health you cannot help others; period. Take care of yourself and you will be much more valuable to others.

Balance- This is life's ultimate challenge; attempt to always keep this in perspective. When times get tough, whether through career, social, or familial challenges, always have your outlet at hand to deal with life's rigors. Exercise, which assist in decreasing stress, is the ultimate keeper of balance in the human body. The more balance you keep, the more positive steps you will be able to take forward. At times it may not be as fast as you like, but these will be firm steps.

Diet- To mean what in terms you are consuming in a given day. This includes all sources of calories, your nutritional plan.

Keep it simple- Is used in this book in regards to what you consume. Do not over complicate food; keep serving sizes for all groups very simplistic in nature so that they work for you.

Creative and flexible- This is used in the context of exercise. You must learn to be creative and flexible in your schedule sometimes to get your regular exercise routine in on a regular basis. Life will throw you curveballs; it is up to you to decide how to hit them!

Transitioning workout- This is the term coined to have very limited work breaks in between larger muscle groups. This is often displayed by utilizing an abdominal exercise as the "rest" period. However, in more advanced stages, a wind sprint or jumping jacks can be rotated in as well.

You are your only measuring stick- This is used in the context that during your life, you must learn to only compare your efforts to yourself and no one else! You are in this battle of life on your own and you can be your own best propeller or worse enemy, the choice is yours!

Sleep cures all- When you think about on a very simplistic level, sleep allows your body to restore itself through many processes. Resting the body is good for the body, mind and soul!

Self-time- This is used in the context of remembering to have your own "dedicated" YOU time. This is where you have the opportunity to completely focus on your physical self. Remember to embed early in life or it will never be a priority to you.

Metabolism is everything- This refers to the points in the book made about ensuring your weight is maintained. Your metabolic rate, the amount of energy (calories) expended while you are at rest, is the most important human body function. Contributing factors to your metabolic rate are exercise and thermic effect of food, which is how many calories it takes for your body to go through the digestive processes of various foods for use and storage.

Documents referred to in Chapters

1. Body mass index table
2. Antioxidants
3. Fruit and vegetable amounts per age and activity level
4. Lean protein list
5. Anatomy of the whole grain
6. Whole grain list
7. Commonly eaten dairy products
8. Healthy fat list
9. ACSM fluid replacement recommendations
10. Basic bodybuilding exercises
11. Home workout basics
12. Abdominal exercises
13. High starch and lower non starch vegetable list
14. Resistance tube exercises
15. US family health plan recommended health screenings for men
16. AHRQ: men stay healthy at any age

You can also determine your BMI using the table below. First, identify your weight (to the nearest 10 pounds) in one of the columns across the top, then move your finger down the column until you come to the row that represents your height. Inside the square where your weight and height meet is a number that is an estimate of your BMI. For example, if you weigh 160 pounds and are 5'7", your BMI is 25.

	WEIGHT															
HEIGHT	**100**	**110**	**120**	**130**	**140**	**150**	**160**	**170**	**180**	**190**	**200**	**210**	**220**	**230**	**240**	**250**
5'0"	20	21	23	25	27	29	31	33	35	37	39	41	43	45	47	49
5'1"	19	21	23	25	26	28	30	32	34	36	38	40	42	43	45	47
5'2"	18	20	22	24	26	27	29	31	33	35	37	38	40	42	44	46
5'3"	18	19	21	23	25	27	28	30	32	34	35	37	39	41	43	44
5'4"	17	19	21	22	24	26	27	29	31	33	34	36	38	39	41	43
5'5"	17	18	20	22	23	25	27	28	30	32	33	35	37	38	40	42
5'6"	16	18	19	21	23	24	26	27	29	31	32	34	36	37	39	40
5'7"	16	17	19	20	22	23	25	27	28	30	31	33	34	36	38	39
5'8"	15	17	18	20	21	23	24	26	27	29	30	32	33	35	36	38
5'9"	15	16	18	19	21	22	24	25	27	28	30	31	32	34	35	37
5'10"	14	16	17	19	20	22	23	24	26	27	29	30	32	33	34	36
5'11"	14	15	17	18	20	21	22	24	25	26	27	28	30	32	33	35
6'0"	14	15	16	18	19	20	22	23	24	26	27	28	30	31	33	34
6'1"	13	15	16	17	18	20	21	22	24	25	26	28	29	30	32	33
6'2"	13	14	15	17	18	19	21	22	23	24	26	27	28	30	31	32
6'3"	12	14	15	16	17	19	20	21	22	24	25	26	27	29	30	31
6'4"	12	13	15	16	17	18	19	21	22	23	24	26	27	28	29	30

Source-http://www.health.harvard.edu/topic/BMI-Calculator
July 4, 2013

Antioxidants

A USDA study analyzed the antioxidant content of *commonly consumed foods*. Researchers tested over 100 foods. Here is a ranked list of the top 20 fruits, vegetables and nuts:

1. Small red bean (dried), 1/2 cup
2. Wild blueberry, 1 cup
3. Red kidney bean (dried), 1/2 cup
4. Pinto bean, 1/2 cup
5. Blueberry (cultivated), 1 cup
6. Cranberry, 1 cup (whole)
7. Artichoke (cooked hearts), 1 cup
8. Blackberry, 1 cup
9. Prune, 1/2 cup
10. Raspberry, 1 cup
11. Strawberry, 1 cup
12. Red delicious apple, 1
13. Granny Smith apple, 1
14. Pecan, 1 ounce
15. Sweet cherry, 1 cup
16. Black plum, 1
17. Russet potato, 1 cooked
18. Black bean (dried), 1/2 cup
19. Plum, 1
20. Gala apple, 1

Sources:

American Chemical Society. "Largest USDA Study Of Food Antioxidants Reveals Best Sources." ScienceDaily 17 June 2004. Halvorsen BL, Holte K, Myhrstad MC, Barikmo I, Hvattum E, Remberg SF, Wold AB, Haffner K, Baugerod H, Andersen LF, Moskaug O, Jacobs DR Jr, Blomhoff R. A Systematic Screening of Total Antioxidants in Dietary Plants. Journal of Nutrition 132:461-471, 2002.

Types of Antioxidants and Food Sources

Antioxidants are abundant in fruits and vegetables, as well as in other foods including nuts, grains, and some meats, poultry, and fish. The list below describes food sources of common antioxidants.

1. Beta-carotene is found in many foods that are orange in color, including sweet potatoes, carrots, cantaloupe, squash, apricots, pumpkin, and mangos. Some green, leafy vegetables, including collard greens, spinach, and kale, are also rich in beta-carotene.

2. Lutein, best known for its association with healthy eyes, is abundant in green, leafy vegetables such as collard greens, spinach, and kale.

3. Lycopene is a potent antioxidant found in tomatoes, watermelon, guava, papaya, apricots, pink grapefruit, blood oranges, and other foods. Estimates suggest 85 percent of American dietary intake of lycopene comes from tomatoes and tomato products.

4. Selenium is a <u>mineral</u>, not an antioxidant <u>nutrient</u>. However, it is a component of antioxidant <u>enzymes</u>. Plant foods like rice and wheat are the major dietary sources of selenium in most countries. The amount of selenium in soil, which varies by region, determines the amount of selenium in the foods grown in that soil. Animals that eat grains or plants grown in selenium-rich soil have higher levels of selenium in their muscle. In the United States, fish, shellfish, red meat, chicken, eggs, garlic, grains (oats and brown rice), wheat germ, and molasses are common sources of dietary selenium. Brazil nuts also contain large quantities of selenium.

5. Vitamin A is found in three main forms: retinol (Vitamin A1), 3,4-

didehydroretinol (Vitamin A2), and 3-hydroxy-retinol (Vitamin A3). Foods rich in vitamin A include liver, sweet potatoes, carrots, squash, broccoli, tomatoes, kale, collards, cantaloupe, peaches, apricots, milk, egg yolks, and mozzarella cheese.

6. Vitamin C is also called ascorbic acid, and can be found in high abundance in many fruits (citrus, like pineapple, orange, lime) mango, papaya, guava, cantaloupe, and vegetables (dark green vegetables like spinach, asparagus, green peppers, brussel sprouts, broccoli, water cress and other greens) red and yellow peppers, tomatoes, tomato juice, and is also found in cereals, beef, poultry, and fish.

7. Vitamin E, also known as alpha-tocopherol, is found in almonds, in many oils including wheat germ, olive, cottonseed, safflower, corn, and soybean oils, and is also found in mangos, nuts, seeds, broccoli, whole grains, legumes and dark leafy vegetables and other foods.

Other Common Antioxidants and food sources

Some common phytochemicals (plant chemicals that have been shown to work just like antioxidants)

• Flavonoids / polyphenols
o soy
o red wine
o purple grapes
o pomegranate
o cranberries
o tea

• Lignan
o flax seed
o oatmeal
o barley
o rye

References
National Cancer Institute- 10/30/12
http://www.cancer.gov/cancertopics/factsheet/preventio
n/antioxidants

1. Blot WJ, Li JY, Taylor PR, et al. Nutrition intervention trials in Linxian, China: supplementation with specific vitamin/mineral combinations, cancer incidence, and disease- specific mortality in the general population. J Natl Cancer Inst 1993;85:1483–91.

2. The Alpha-Tocopherol, Beta Carotene Cancer Prevention Study Group. The effects of vitamin E and beta carotene on the incidence of lung cancer and other cancers in male smokers. N Engl J Med 1994;330:1029–35.

3. Omenn GS, Goodman G, Thomquist M, et al. The beta-carotene and retinol efficacy trial (CARET) for chemoprevention of lung cancer in high risk populations: smokers and asbestos-exposed workers. Cancer Res 1994;54(7 Suppl):2038s–43s.

4.   Hennekens CH, Buring JE, Manson JE, Stampfer M, Rosner B, Cook NR, et al. Lack of effect of long-term supplementation with beta carotene on the incidence of malignant neoplasms and cardiovascular disease. N Engl J Med 1996;334:1145–9.

5.   Lee IM, Cook NR, Manson JE. Beta-carotene supplementation and incidence of cancer and cardiovascular disease: Women's Health Study. J Natl Cancer Inst 1999;91:2102–6.

6.   Cleveland Clinic -10/30/12
http://my.clevelandclinic.org/heart/prevention/askdi
etician/ask6_01.aspx

Fruit and Vegetable Amounts per age and activity level

Men

Activity Level	Age	Fruits	Vegetables
Less Active	19-50	2 Cups	3 Cups
Less Active	51+	2 Cups	2.5 Cups
Moderately Active	19-30	2 Cups	3.5 Cups
Moderately Active	31+	2 Cups	3 Cups
Active	19-30	2.5 Cups	4 Cups
Active	31-50	2.5 Cups	3.5 Cups
Active	51+	2 Cups	3 Cups

Source- http://www.fruitsandveggiesmorematters.org/wp-content/uploads/UserFiles/File/pdf/resources/cdc/HowMany_Brochure.pdf
10/30/12

Lean Protein List

All meats (animal flesh) should be approximately palm-sized after cooking for one serving. All meats should be baked, broiled, grilled, stir- fried, rotisserie, or lightly sautéed.

- Chicken (breast is leanest)
- Turkey (breast is leanest)
- Turkey based products (should come from the turkey breast-read ingredients)
- Pork (try cuts like loin or round)
- Beef (try cuts like loin or round)
- Ground meats (use 93% or leaner)
- Fish (to begin all types)
- All Wild Game (i.e. Venison, Ostrich, or Buffalo/Bison)
- Egg Whites or Substitutes (per RD Recommendation) Typical Male serving is 6-9 egg whites, typical Female serving is 4-6 egg whites.
- Soy based products
- Whey based products (i.e. protein shakes) typically 1-2 scoops= 1 serving. Typical male serving is 2 scoops
- Fat free or 1% dairy products

Anatomy of the Whole Grain

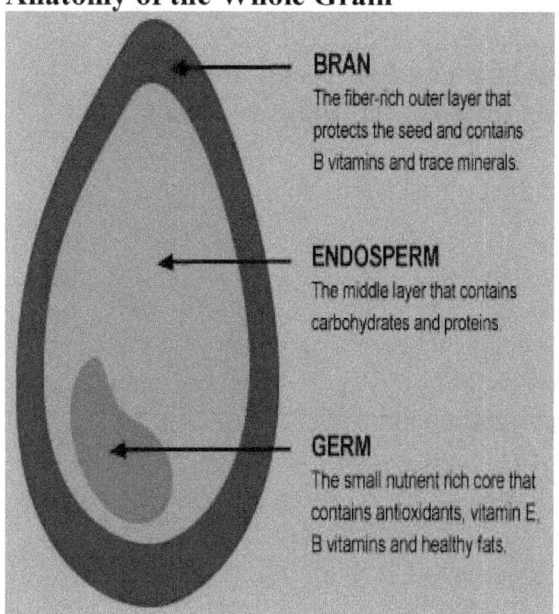

BRAN

The fiber-rich outer layer that protects the seed and contains B vitamins and trace minerals.

ENDOSPERM

The middle layer that contains carbohydrates and proteins.

GERM

The small nutrient rich core that contains antioxidants, vitamin E, B vitamins and healthy fats.

When grains are milled, or refined, the bran and germ are removed, leaving only the endosperm.

Source- http://wholegrainnation.eatbetteramerica.com/facts/
10/30/12

Whole Grain List

All Whole grain servings should be based on ½ cup unless otherwise noted on package. At least 1-2 servings per day.

• Whole Grain Bread (light bread recommended, no more than 50 calories per slice)
• Brown or Wild rice
• Whole oats, steel-cut or rolled
• Whole grain noted dry cereal such as Cheerios or Total
• Whole wheat berries, whole wheat bulgur, whole wheat couscous and other strains of wheat such as kamut and spelt
• Whole rye
• Hulled barley (pot, scotch, and pearled barley often have much of their bran removed)
• Triticale (pronounced tri-ti-kay-lee)
• Millet
• Teff (reported to be the world's smallest grain and to have a sweet, malt-like flavor)
• Buckwheat, quinoa (pronounced keen- wah), and amarant

Commonly eaten dairy products

*Be careful of excess calories and limit choices
In general, 1 cup of milk, yogurt, or soymilk (soy beverage), 1 ½ ounces of natural cheese, or 2 ounces of processed cheese can be considered as 1 cup from the Dairy Group. Three (3) cups equivalent are suggested per day for every age group; ensure either fat free (FF) or low fat (1%) are selected.

Milk- 1 cup=serving size
Fat-free (skim) Low fat
(1%) Chocolate*
Strawberry*

Milk-based desserts*- 1 cup=serving size
Puddings (FF or 1%) Ice milk (FF or
1%) Frozen yogurt (FF or 1%) Ice
cream (FF or 1%)

Calcium-fortified soymilk-1 cup=serving size
(soy beverage)

Cheese*- 1.5 ounce=serving size
Hard natural cheeses
Cheddar Mozzarella
Swiss Parmesan

Soft cheeses*
Ricotta- ½ cup=serving size
Cottage cheese-2 cups=serving size

Processed cheeses*- 2 ounces= serving size
American

Yogurt-1 cup=serving size
Fat-free
Low fat

Source- http://www.choosemyplate.gov/food-groups/dairy.html
10/30/12

Healthy fat list
Fats that are higher in mono and polyunsaturated fats.

Avocado
Sunflower seeds
Pumpkin seeds
Natural peanut butter or other nut butters
Low-sodium nuts
Olives and olive oil
Safflower oil
Canola oil
Sunflower oil
Flax seed oil

ACSM Fluid Replacement Recommendations

Proper hydration is important for optimal physical performance and endurance. Because both dehydration and over hydration can be a serious problem for athletes, experts at the American College of Sports Medicine (ACSM) regularly update their position paper recommendations for fluid replacement for physical activity. According to the ACSM, because hydration needs can vary considerably between individuals, and for the same individual under different environmental conditions and different physical activities, it's important for athletes to develop a personalized hydration plan. Highlights from the 2007 ACSM fluid replacement recommendations:

- **Individuals can monitor their hydration status by employing simple urine and body weight measurements**. Several days of first morning body weights can be used to establish base-line body weights that represent "normal" body water levels. Body weight changes can reflect sweat losses during exercise and can be used to calculate individual fluid replacement needs for specific exercise and environmental conditions.

- **Fluid replacement before exercise, if needed, is meant to start the physical activity at "normal" body water and electrolyte levels**. Fluid should be consumed several hours before exercise to enable fluid absorption and to allow urine output to return to normal levels. ACSM recommends consuming beverages with sodium and/or salted snacks to help stimulate thirst or retain fluids.

- **Fluid replacement during exercise is meant to prevent excessive dehydration (weight loss greater than two percent from baseline body weight) and to avoid excessive changes in electrolyte balance in order to avert compromised performance.** The amount and rate of fluid replacement will depend on the individual and the activity, accounting for the opportunity to drink. Exercise- associated hyponatremia, which can occur in endurance events, is associated primarily with consuming fluid in excess of sweating rate. Individuals should develop customized fluid replacement programs that prevent excessive dehydration as well as over hydration. The routine measurement of pre- and post-exercise body weights is useful for determining sweat rates and customized fluid replacement programs. The guidelines note that consuming beverages containing electrolytes and carbohydrates often provides more benefits than consuming water alone. Learn how to calculate your sweat rate.

- **Fluid replacement after exercise is meant to fully replace any fluid and electrolyte losses.** If time permits, regular meals and beverages will restore normal hydration levels. Consuming beverages and snacks with sodium will help expedite rapid and complete recovery by stimulating thirst and fluid retention. Individuals needing rapid and complete recovery from excessive dehydration can drink ~1.5 L of fluid for each kilogram of body weight lost.

Reference

Exercise and Fluid Replacement Position Stand, American College of Sports Medicine, Med Sci Sports Exer. 2007:39;377-390.

Basic Bodybuilding Exercises

*Will denote the most bang for your buck in my opinion if you are time limited!

Chest
• Push up- varying arm widths
• *Dumbbell or Barbell press- varying angles to reach your upper, mid and lower chest
• Chest press- this can be a machine or a weight plate loaded machine
• *Dips

Back
• *Pull up- varying arm widths/grips
• Pull down- machine or weight plate loaded machine
• Low Row- machine or weight plate loaded machine or barbell
• T-Bar Row- weight plate loaded
• Dumbbell row
• Dumbbell pullovers
• *Deadlifts
• Hyperextensions

Shoulders
• *Dumbbell press
• *Front barbell press
• *Dumbbell or Barbell Shrugs
• Rear Deltoid machine or dumbbell movement
• Side Deltoid machine or dumbbell movement
• Front dumbbell or barbell raises

Legs
• *Squat- barbell or machine or dumbbell
• *Leg Press
• Leg Extension
• Leg Curl

- Abductor/Adductor machine
- Calve raises or machine

Triceps
- *Close grip bench press
- *Dips
- Tricep extension
- Reverse grip tricep pushdown

Biceps
- *Dumbbell or barbell curl
- *Seated dumbbell curl
- Preacher curl
- Concentration curl
- Machine or cable curl

Abdominals
- *Leg raises- varying degrees and types such as Roman Chair raises
- *Crunches- using slant board- varying angles
- Abdominal machines

Home Workout Basics

The following is my personal opinion of best value home equipment when space is limited.

Resistance *= MUSTS; others are optional if you have the space and finances
- *Dumbbells- purchase the dumbbells that can be dialed to the weight that you prefer. I would suggest dialed weights from 10-90 pounds.
- *Multi-position bench- I prefer a five or seven position bench
- *Exercise ball- check your height to ensure correct ball purchased
- Bosu Ball
- Pushup bars
- Pull up bar
- *Resistance tubes- one or two with varying strengths
- All in one pull up/dip rack
- Smith machine- with up to 200 pound of free weights

Cardiovascular equipment *= MUSTS; others are optional if you have the space and finances
- Treadmill or tread climber
- Scaled down rowing machine (low impact on most joints)
- Stationary Bike (low impact on most joints)
- Elliptical machine (low impact on most joints)
- *Running sneakers (for outdoors)

Abdominal Exercises

*Advanced movements
Some movements noted below can also be accomplished with BOSU ball instead of stability/physio ball.
As you progress and you have the access to, you can move towards more resistance movements which are typically found in your local gym.
Descriptions of all exercises can easily be found on the internet

Lower
Reverse crunch/lower abdominal crunch
Leg lift/leg raises
Flutter kicks
Stability/physio ball leg crunches
*Stability/physio ball piques
*Hanging leg raises/Roman chair

Middle
Standard abdominal crunch Standard sit ups Stability/physio ball crunches
*Stability/physio ball roll in crunches
*Hanging leg raises/Roman chair

Sides
Bicycle crunches
Knee ups
Side leg raises
*Hanging leg raises/Roman chair
*Side planks

Overall
Planks- all types- stability/physio ball as well
Double crunch

High Starch (complex carbohydrate) and Lower or non-Starch Vegetables

High Starch (complex carbohydrate)
- Potatoes
- Corn
- Parsnip
- Pumpkin
- Squash
- Yams and sweet potatoes
- Pinto beans
- Garbanzo beans
- Lentils
- Peas
- Lima beans

Low or non-starchy vegetables
- Spinach
- Turnip greens
- Beet greens
- Kale
- Mustard greens
- Amaranth greens
- Lettuce
- Broccoli
- Green beans
- Cabbage
- Cucumbers
- Peas
- Green peppers
- Brussels sprouts
- Artichokes
- Leeks
- Scallion
- Zucchini
- Yellow and orange peppers

- Yellow squash
- Carrots
- Yellow tomatoes
- Rutabagas
- Tomatoes
- Beets
- Red peppers
- Red cabbage
- Radishes
- Rhubarb
- Jicama
- Onions
- Cauliflower
- Turnips
- Mushrooms

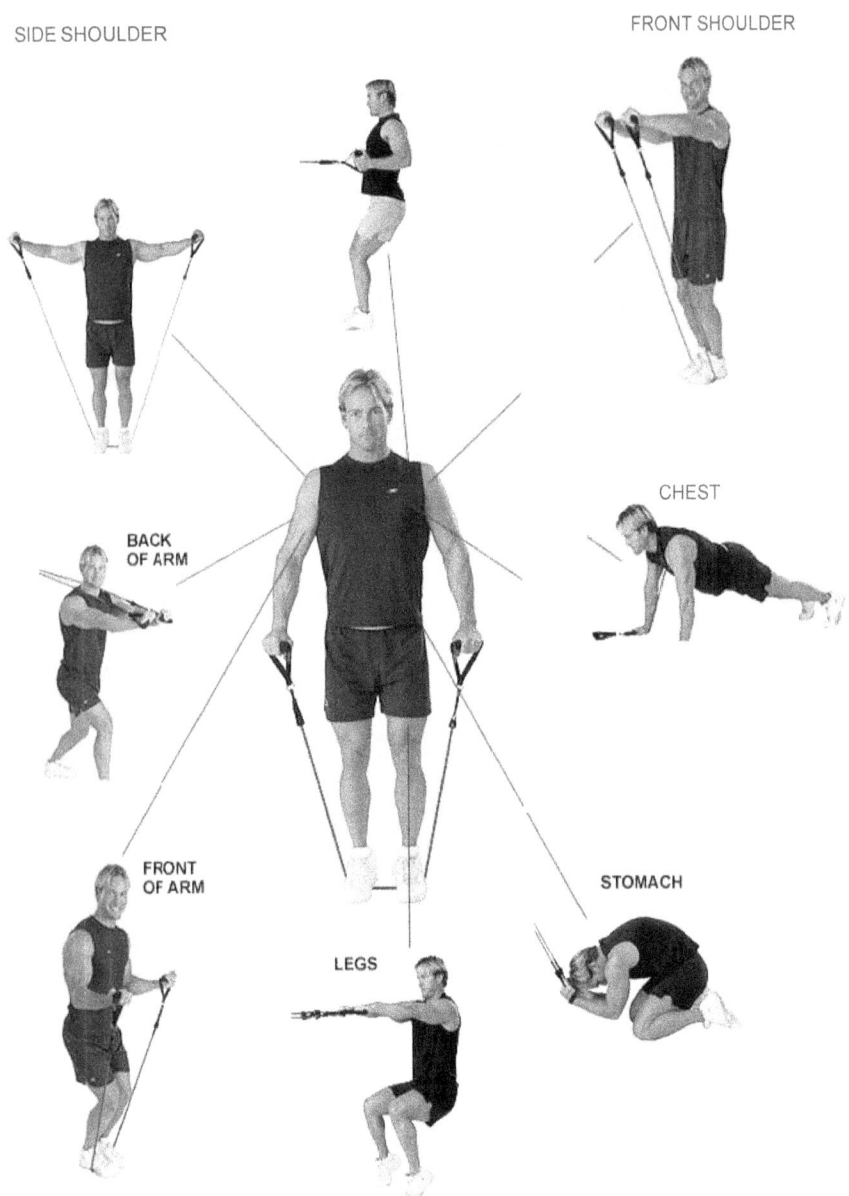

BACK

SIDE SHOULDER

FRONT SHOULDER

CHEST

BACK
OF ARM

FRONT
OF ARM

STOMACH

LEGS

Recommended Health Screenings for Men US Family Health Plan strongly encourages all of its members to get regular preventive health screenings. The chart below gives some guidelines for preventive health screenings for men. Be sure to request and discuss these recommendations with your Primary Care Provider (PCP). Depending on personal risk factors and family medical history, your PCP may recommend additional or more frequent screenings. **EXAM**	STARTING AGE	FREQ.
Routine Physical Exam (Preventive health visit)	18 40 50	Every 3 – 5 years Every 1 – 2 years Annual
CANCER SCREENING		
Colon Cancer Fecal occult blood test, Colonoscopy *or* Sigmoidoscopy	50 50 50	Annual* Every 10 years* Every 3 – 5 years*
Prostate Digital rectal exam PSA (blood test)	50 (earlier if family history or if African-American) 50 (earlier if family history or if African-American)	Annual Annual
Skin Cancer	18	Self-exam monthly Clinical exam by healthcare provider every 3 years*
Testicular	13	Self-exam monthly and Clinical exam by Healthcare provider at preventative health visit

HEART HEALTH

Abdominal Aortic Aneurysm (AAA)	65 – 75	One time screening for men with history of smoking
Blood Pressure	18	Every visit or at least every 1 – 2 years
Cholesterol (blood test)	18	Every 5 years

OTHER RECOMMENDED SCREENINGS

Diabetes (blood test)	18	Every 3 years*
Weight/Body Mass Index	18	At preventive health visit

INFECTIOUS DISEASE SCREENINGS

Hepatitis C	18, if high risk	Discuss with your provider
HIV	13, especially if high risk	Discuss with your provider
STD's (Sexually transmitted infections)	18 (or earlier if sexually active)	Discuss with your provider
Tuberculosis	18, if high risk	Annual

SENSORY SCREENINGS

Eye Exam	18 At any age if diabetic	Every 2 years, Annual if diabetic
Hearing	18 50	Every 10 yrs Every 3 yrs
Oral and Dental Exam**	Starting in childhood	1 – 2 times a year
IMMUNIZATIONS	18	Discuss with your provider
BEHAVIORAL HEALTH	18	Discuss with your provider

Resources:
• MedlinePlus (www.nlm.nih.gov/medlineplus/)
• TRICARE (www.tricare.mil
• US Department of Health and Human Services/Centers for Disease Control
and Prevention (www.cdc.gov)
* Depending on personal risk factors and family medical history, your PCP
may recommend additional or more frequent screenings.
** Dental care is not a covered benefit; however, all individuals are strongly encouraged to practice good dental health and hygiene. A complete oral cavity exam should be part of the routine preventive health performed by your PCP.
Recommended Health Screenings for Men, last updated 2/2010.

Men: Stay Healthy at Any Age

Use the information in this pamphlet to help you stay healthy. Learn about which screening tests to get, whether you need medicines to prevent diseases, and steps you can take for good health.

Get the Screenings You Need

Screenings are tests that look for diseases before you have symptoms. Blood pressure checks and tests for high cholesterol are examples of screenings.

You can get some screenings, such as blood pressure readings, in your doctor's office. Others such as colonoscopy, a test for colorectal cancer, need special equipment, so you may need to go to a different office.

After a screening test, ask when you will see the results and who you should talk to about them.

Abdominal Aortic Aneurysm

If you are between the ages of 65 and 75 and have ever been a smoker, talk to your doctor or nurse about being screened for abdominal aortic aneurysm (AAA). AAA is a bulging in your abdominal aorta, the largest artery in your body. An AAA may burst, which can cause dangerous bleeding and death.

Colorectal Cancer

Have a screening test for colorectal cancer starting at age 50. If you have a family history of colorectal cancer, you may need to be screened earlier. Several different tests can detect this cancer. Your doctor can help you decide which is best for you.

Depression

Your emotional health is as important as your physical health. Talk to your doctor or nurse about being screened for depression especially if during the last 2 weeks:

- You have felt down, sad, or hopeless.
- You have felt little interest or pleasure in doing things.

Diabetes

Get screened for diabetes if your blood pressure is higher than 135/80 or if you take medication for high blood pressure. Diabetes (high blood sugar) can cause problems with your heart, brain, eyes, feet, kidneys, nerves, and other body parts.

High Blood Pressure

Starting at age 18, have your blood pressure checked at least every 2 years. High blood pressure is 140/90 or higher. High blood pressure can cause strokes, heart attacks, kidney and eye problems, and heart failure.

High Cholesterol

If you are 35 or older, have your cholesterol checked. Have your cholesterol checked starting at age 20 if:

- You use tobacco.
- You are obese.
- You have diabetes or high blood pressure.
- You have a personal history of heart disease or blocked arteries.
- A man in your family had a heart attack before age 50 or a woman, before age 60.

HIV

Talk with your health care team about HIV screening if any of these apply to you:

- You have had unprotected sex with multiple partners.
- You have sex with men.
- You use or have used injection drugs.
- You exchange sex for money or drugs or have sex partners who do.
- You have or had a sex partner who is HIV-infected or injects drugs.
- You are being treated for a sexually transmitted disease.
- You had a blood transfusion between 1978 and 1985.
- You have any other concerns.

Syphilis

Ask your doctor or nurse whether you should be screened for syphilis.

Overweight and Obesity

The best way to learn if you are overweight or obese is to find your body mass index (BMI). You can find your BMI by entering your height and weight into a BMI calculator, such as the one available at: http://www.nhlbisupport.com/bmi/

A BMI between 18.5 and 25 indicates a normal weight. Persons with a BMI of 30 or higher may be obese.

If you are obese, talk to your doctor or nurse about seeking intensive counseling and getting help with changing your behaviors to lose weight. Overweight and obesity can lead to diabetes and cardiovascular disease.

It's Your Body!

You know your body better than anyone else. Always tell your doctor or nurse about any changes in your health, including your vision and hearing. Ask them about being checked for any condition you are concerned about, not just the ones here. If you are wondering about diseases such as prostate cancer or skin cancer, for example, ask about them.

Take Preventive Medicines If You Need Them
Aspirin

If you are 45 or older, ask your doctor if you should take aspirin to prevent heart disease.

Immunizations

- Get a flu shot every year.
- If you are 65 or older, get a pneumonia shot.
- Depending on health problems, you may need a pneumonia shot at a younger age or need shots to prevent diseases like whooping cough or shingles.
- Talk with your doctor or nurse about whether you need vaccinations. You can also find which ones you need by going to:

http://www.cdc.gov/vaccines/recs/schedules/default.htm.
Source- http://www.ahrq.gov/patients-consumers/patient-

involvement/healthy-men/healthy-men.html
July 4, 2013.

Appendix of web links used in book

http://www.nhlbi.nih.gov/guidelines/obesity/bmi_tbl.pdf
http://www.cdc.gov/men/lcod/2006/AllMales2006.pdf
http://wholegrainnation.eatbetteramerica.com/facts/
http://www.choosemyplate.gov/foodgroups/vegetables.html
http://www.choosemyplate.gov/foodgroups/fruits.html
http://www.choosemyplate.gov/foodgroups/proteinfoods.html
http://www.choosemyplate.gov/foodgroups/grains.html
http://www.choosemyplate.gov/foodgroups/grains.html
http://www.choosemyplate.gov/foodgroups/dairy.html

About the Author

Joseph V. Gennusa III, PhD, RDN, LDN is currently a Research Study Director at Johns Hopkins University in Baltimore, Maryland. A Registered Dietitian for over the past fifteen years; whose career and personal focus is on optimal longevity. He has a passion for the equilibrium in life between the physical, mental and spiritual state of the human body. He has and understands the dedicated mind of the athlete and thus is what drove him through his graduate and doctoral work and led his career to evolve to current. Many years in the beginning of his career had been spent educating on cardiovascular, diabetes, and obesity management. For many years he contributed at the state level through directing senior nutrition and health promotion programs. He continues his current work in disparity research assisting those with serious mental illness to reduce cardiovascular disease risk through lifestyle interventions.

Joe practices what he preaches as he is a steadfast and dedicated believer in this book! It is if you say, "tried and tested" by Joe as he is in his fourth decade of life. He will certainly do his best to follow the next chapters in his life.